The Sexual Secrets

In this book you will learn to

Have multiple orgasms without losing your erection

Experience longer, more intense whole-body orgasms

Use your sexual energy to improve your overall health

Increase your sexual energy and vitality

Recognize the signs of your partner's desire

Help your partner to become multi-orgasmic

Master thrusting techniques that will completely satisfy your partner

Use sexuality to deepen your spirituality

Make all sex safer

End premature ejaculation

Overcome impotence

Increase the size and strength of your penis

Raise your sperm count

Prevent and help prostate problems

Increase your sexual strength in middle and older age

Maintain the passion in your relationship as you age together

THE

Sexual Secrets

MULTI-

Every Man

ORGASMIC

Should Know

MAN

Mantak Chia and

Douglas Abrams Arava

HarperSanFrancisco
An Imprint of HarperCollins*Publishers*

■ A TREE CLAUSE BOOK

HarperSanFrancisco and the authors, in association with The Basic Foundation,
a not-for-profit organization whose primary mission is reforestation, will facilitate
the planting of two trees for every one tree used in the manufacture of this book.

HarperCollins Web Site: http://www.harpercollins.com

HarperCollins®, ■®, HarperSanFrancisco™, and A TREE CLAUSE BOOK®
are trademarks of HarperCollins Publishers Inc.

FIRST HARPERCOLLINS PAPERBACK EDITION PUBLISHED IN 1997
Illustrations by Todd Buck
Book design by Ralph Fowler
Set in Fairfield Light and Frutiger

Library of Congress Cataloging-in-Publication Data
Chia, Mantak
The multi-orgasmic man : sexual secrets every man should know /
Mantak Chia and Douglas Abrams Arava. — 1st ed.
Includes bibliographical references.
ISBN 0–06–251335–4 (cloth)
ISBN 0–06–251336–2 (pbk.)
1. Sex instruction for men.   2. Men—Sexual behavior.
3. Sex—Religious aspects—Taoism.   4. Orgasm.
I. Arava, Douglas Abrams.   II. Title.
HQ36.C424   1996
613.9'6'081—dc20   95–51976

05 04 03   ❖ RRDH   30 29 28

For our sons, Max and Jesse

CHAPTER EIGHT

Before You Call the Plumber   182

CHAPTER NINE

Making Love for a Lifetime   204

WARNING *This is not just another sex book.* There is so much talk about sex today, and yet still so much misunderstanding, that it is difficult to know what is of any value or use. You have no doubt seen advertisements from sexperts that promise to teach you how to become the world's greatest lover, have daylong orgasms, and reach sexual ecstasy—all without doing anything. Because this book is based on a three-thousand-year tradition of actual sexual experience, the authors are well aware of the effort that is involved—pleasurable as it may be—in changing your sex life. Learning sexual secrets is one thing, but using them is quite another. The techniques in this book have been tested and refined by countless lovers over thousands of years in the laboratory of real life. We have tried to present them in as clear and simple a way as possible, but the only way to benefit from them is to really use them.

These are powerful practices. The techniques given in this book can profoundly improve your health as well as your sexuality. However, we do not give any diagnoses or suggestions for medication. People who have high blood pressure, heart disease, or a generally weak condition should proceed slowly in the practice. If you have a medical condition, a medical doctor should be consulted. If you have questions about or difficulty with the practice, you should contact a Healing Tao instructor in your area (see the appendix: "Healing Tao Books and Instructors").

We would like to acknowledge all of the multi-orgasmic men and women from around the world who contributed to this book with their candid descriptions of their experience and their sexual practice. The quotes that appear in this book are taken directly from interviews and questionnaires and have been edited only for clarity and readability in English. We would especially like to thank the gifted Healing Tao instructors who contributed to this book with their wisdom, their experience, their humor, and their friendship— Michael Winn, Marcia Kerwit, B. J. Santerre, Masahiro Ouchi, Angela Shen, Louis Shen, Walter Beckley, Stefan Siegrist, and Karl Danskin—as well as numerous others who have worked over the years to simplify and perfect the techniques offered here. We would also like to thank the sexologists whose pioneering work has expanded our understanding of male multiple orgasms and human sexual pleasure, especially William Hartman and Marilyn Fithian, Bernie Zilbergeld, Marion Dunn, Alan and Donna Brauer, Beverly Whipple, Alice Kahn Ladis, John Perry, Lonnie Barbach, Barbara Keesling, and of course Alfred Kinsey and William Masters and Virginia Johnson. In addition, we would like to acknowledge the numerous scholars and students of Taoism who have contributed to our knowledge of Sexual Kung Fu, including Douglas Wile, whose masterful *Art of the Bedchamber* served as the source for most of the translations in this book. And Megory Anderson, for everything.

We would like to thank our gifted agent, Heide Lange, whose experience, insight, and warmth were an endless source of encouragement during the writing of this book, and our excellent editor, John Loudon, who believed in and helped develop the book from the very beginning. We would also like to thank the rest of the people at Harper San Francisco, who have helped shepherd and shape the book through the publishing process and into the world— especially Karen Levine, Joel Fotinos, Rosana Francescato, Carl Walesa, Ralph Fowler, Laura Beers, and Peter Evers.

Most of all we would like to thank our life partners and coauthors, Maneewan Chia and Rachel Carlton Arava, who have taught us the real secret and the true meaning of the Tao.

Over three thousand years ago, the Chinese recognized that men can achieve multiple orgasms by delaying and even withholding ejaculation. This is possible because orgasm and ejaculation are two distinct physical processes, though they have long been equated in the West. Although clearly less precise than today's sex researchers, the ancient Chinese recorded their findings in detail for future generations of sexual and spiritual seekers.[1]

In the West, it was not until the 1940s that pioneering sex researcher Alfred Kinsey reported similar discoveries.[2] Yet even several decades later, after his claims have been proved repeatedly in the laboratory, most men remain unaware of their multi-orgasmic potential. Without this knowledge and without a clear technique, men are unable to feel the difference between the crescendo of orgasm and the crash of ejaculation.

Male sexuality in the West remains incorrectly focused on the inevitably disappointing goal of ejaculation ("getting off") instead of the orgasmic process of lovemaking. *The Multi-Orgasmic Man* shows men how to separate orgasm and ejaculation in their own bodies, allowing them to transform the momentary release of ejaculation into countless peaks of whole-body orgasms. In the words of one multi-orgasmic man, "In the normal, everyday sort of ejaculation my pleasure is quickly over with. Not so in multiple orgasms. The pleasure generated here stays with me throughout the day. There seems to be no final peak to this pleasure, either. This practice offers the added bonus of affording extra energy, so I am just never tired. Now I can have as much sex as I want and I can control it rather than have it control me. What more can a man ask for?"

The Multi-Orgasmic Man also shows men how to satisfy the multi-orgasmic potential of their partners. One multi-orgasmic man who had been practicing the techniques in this book for three months explained his experience: "Basically, I have slept with three women since starting to practice these techniques, and *all three* have told me that I was their best, literally said it to me while we were in bed: 'This is the best I have ever had.'"

Women who read *The Multi-Orgasmic Man* will learn secrets about male sexuality that few women, and even few men, know. Couples who read it together will find levels of sexual ecstasy and satisfaction that they may never have imagined were possible. As one partner of a multi-orgasmic man put it, "Our lovemaking has always been good, but now it is so much richer and more balanced with both of us experiencing many waves of orgasm. Multi-orgasms, though, are just the beginning of the profound changes that this practice has made in our relationship. Our love is much deeper and more intimate now."

The fact that men can have multiple orgasms is so surprising to most of us that we may find it hard to believe. It is worth remembering that only in the last forty years have female multiple orgasms been recognized and accepted as "normal." Even more surprising is the number of women who have become multi-orgasmic—once they were told it was possible. Since the fifties, when Kinsey was studying female sexuality, the number of women who experience multiple orgasms has tripled, from 14 percent to over 50 percent![3] In the 1980s, sexologists William Hartman and Marilyn Fithian found that 12 percent of the men they studied were multi-orgasmic. As men recognize that they also have this potential and learn some simple techniques, more and more of them will discover that they too can experience multiple orgasms.

In this book we draw on both ancient Taoist (pronounced *DOW-ist*) practices and the most recent scientific knowledge to show you how to separate orgasm from ejaculation, how to experience multiple orgasms, and how to improve your overall health. The Taoists were originally a group of seekers in ancient China (around 500 B.C.E.) who were extremely interested in health and spirituality. Although many of the sexual techniques they developed are now more than two thousand years old, they are as effective today as they were then. Since the techniques in this book were introduced to the West fifteen years ago, there has been a quiet sexual revolution going on among ordinary men who have tried these techniques and proved that they work. However, we believe that the only real proof is in your own body. We hope you will accept or reject the information given here based on your own experience.

Multiple orgasms are not just for adolescent boys, unusually lucky older men, or religious adepts. A software salesman in his thirties who calls himself a "cynical, uptight New Yorker" sat down one evening with the exercises in this book and had six orgasms: "The orgasms got more powerful one after the other. It was like nothing I had ever experienced. But the most amazing thing is that I had been working too much and was getting sick. The next morning I woke up healthy and with more energy than I can remember." According to Taoist sexuality, experiencing multiple orgasms without ejaculating can also help men achieve their body's optimum health and even, believe it or not, live longer.

Taoist sexuality, also called Sexual Kung Fu, began as a branch of Chinese medicine. (*Kung fu* literally means "practice," so *Sexual Kung Fu* simply means "sexual practice.") The ancient Taoists were themselves doctors and were concerned as much with the body's physical well-being as with its sexual satisfaction. Sexual Kung Fu helps men increase their vitality and longevity by allowing them to avoid the fatigue and depletion that follow ejaculation—to stop them from, literally, going to seed.

In chapter 1, we describe the Eastern and Western evidence for male multiple orgasms. We also discuss recent scientific research that seems to confirm the ancient Taoist understanding about the importance of orgasming without ejaculating. In reporting on these surprising studies, the *New York Times* concluded, "Creating sperm is far more difficult than scientists had imagined, demanding a diversion of resources that might otherwise go into assuring a male's long-term health."[4]

Theory without practice, however, is worthless. So in chapters 2 and 3 we give you the "solo practice" that you can use to develop your multi-orgasmic ability—whether you have a partner or not. Many men begin experiencing multiple orgasms within a week or two, and most are able to master the technique within three to six months.

Chapters 4 and 5 teach you the "duo practice" that you will use to share Sexual Kung Fu with a partner and to pleasure her in ways she probably never imagined were possible.

Although women will benefit from reading the entire book, chapter 6 is written especially for them and explains what they will need to know to help their partners—and themselves—reach their multi-orgasmic potential.

Chapter 7 is written for gay men and describes the specific practices they need to learn for a satisfying and healthy multi-orgasmic sex life.

Chapter 8 addresses the concerns of men who are experiencing difficulties with their sexuality, such as premature ejaculation, impotence, and infertility. Taoist sexuality offers completely different ways to think about and overcome these problems.

Finally, chapter 9 offers advice on how men and their partners can have a lifetime of ecstatic sexual intimacy. It begins with a section for middle-aged and older men, who often experience a decline in their sexual appetite and potency. We present research on multi-orgasmic men that contradicts the widely held belief that male sexuality peaks in the teens and declines slowly thereafter. The Taoists have always known that if a man understands the true nature of his sexuality, it will only improve as he matures. This chapter also includes a section on how we can help our sons begin a life of healthy and satisfying sexuality. If only *our* fathers had known!

China produced the world's first, most comprehensive, and most detailed sex manuals. In *The Multi-Orgasmic Man* we continue this long tradition by providing men and their partners with a practical, straightforward guide to transforming their sexuality. Although in Taoism sexuality and spirituality are not separated, we realize that some readers will be interested exclusively in practical sexual advice and that others will want to learn more about the sacred dimension of their sexuality. Starting with basic techniques that all readers will need in order to become multi-orgasmic, we gradually add more subtle techniques for readers who are interested in using their sexuality as a path to improving their health and deepening their spirituality.

It is worth mentioning that this is not a book about Taoism, either as a philosophy or as a religion. (One of the authors of this book, Mantak Chia, has already written over ten books that explain in great detail the practical teachings of this ancient tradition, from which he has developed a comprehensive health system called the Healing Tao.) In *The Multi-Orgasmic Man,* we offer practical Taoist techniques that have been confirmed by scientific study to readers who are looking not for a new religious system but for a deeper experience of their own sexuality.

It is also our hope that this book will spark further scientific research to confirm or revise the theory and practice offered here. We believe that the time for secrecy and cultural chauvinism has passed. East and West can share their knowledge for the benefit of all modern lovers who seek sexual fulfillment in this age of carnal confusion.

The Proof Is in Your Pants

You may already have experienced multiple orgasms. Surprising as this may sound, many men are multi-orgasmic before they enter adolescence and begin to ejaculate: Kinsey's research suggested that more than half of all preadolescent boys were able to reach a second orgasm within a short period of time and nearly a third were able to achieve five or more orgasms one after the other. This led Kinsey to argue that "climax is clearly possible without ejaculation."

But multiple orgasms are not just limited to prepubescent boys. Kinsey continues: "There are older males, even in their thirties and older, who are able to equal this performance." In *Fundamentals of Human Sexuality,* Dr. Herant Katchadourian adds: "Some men are able to inhibit the emission of semen while they experience the orgasmic contractions: in other words they have nonejaculatory orgasms. Such orgasms do not seem to be followed by a refractory period [loss of erection], thereby allowing these men to have consecutive or multiple orgasms like women."

Why do most men lose their ability to be multi-orgasmic? It is possible that for many men the experience of ejaculating, when it happens, is so overwhelming that it eclipses the experience of orgasm and causes men to lose the ability to distinguish between the two. One multi-orgasmic man described the first time he ejaculated: "I still remember it clearly. There I was orgasming as usual, but this time a white liquid came spurting out. I thought I was dying. I swore to God that I would never masturbate again—which of course lasted about a day." Since orgasm and ejaculation generally occur within seconds of one another, it is easy to confuse them.[1] To become multi-orgasmic, you must learn (or possibly relearn) the ability to separate the different sensations of arousal and to revel in orgasm without cresting over into ejaculation. Understanding how orgasm and ejaculation are different will help you distinguish the two in your own body.

Brain Waves and Reflexes

Orgasm is one of the most intense and satisfying human experiences, and if you have ever had an orgasm—and almost all men have—you will not need to have it defined. All orgasms, however, are not created equal. Orgasm is slightly different for each person and even different for the same person at different times. Nonetheless, men's orgasms share certain characteristics, including rhythmic body movements, increased heart rate, muscle tension, and then a sudden release of tension, including pelvic contractions. They feel good, too. After noting that "orgasm is the least understood of the sexual processes," the thirteenth edition of *Smith's General Urology* explains that orgasm includes "involuntary rhythmic contractions of the anal sphincter, hyperventilation [increased breathing rate], tachycardia [increased heart rate], and elevation of blood pressure."

These definitions include changes that occur throughout your entire body. However, for a long time orgasm was seen—and for many men is still seen—as strictly a genital affair. In the West, Wilhelm Reich, in his controversial book *The Function of Orgasm,* was the first to argue that orgasm involved the whole body and not just the genitals.[2] In the East, the Taoists have long known that orgasm could be a whole-body experience and developed techniques for expanding orgasmic pleasure.

Many sex researchers are now arguing that orgasm really has more to do with our brain than our brawn. Brain-wave research is beginning to reveal that orgasm may occur primarily in the brain. That you can have an orgasm in your sleep—without any bodily touch—seems to confirm this theory. Further support comes from neurologist Robert J. Heath of Tulane University, who discovered that when certain parts of the brain are stimulated with electrodes they produce sexual pleasure identical to that produced by physical stimulation. Many sex therapists are fond of saying that sex takes place in the brain. There is some truth to this statement—especially when it comes to orgasm.

Unlike orgasm, which is a peak emotional and physical experience, ejaculation is simply a reflex that occurs at the base of the spine and results in the ejection of semen. Michael Winn, senior Healing Tao instructor and coauthor of *Taoist Secrets of Love: Cultivating Male Sexual Energy,* explains: "A lot of men are freaked out by the very idea of nonejaculatory orgasm because they've been having ejaculatory sex for such a long time, often decades. So the first thing to do is demystify ejaculation, which is just an involuntary muscle spasm."

With practice, you can learn to experience the peak feeling of orgasm without triggering the reflex of ejaculation. In the next two chapters we will explain, step-by-step, exactly how to separate orgasm from ejaculation and how to expand your orgasms throughout your body. But first let's look at the evidence that men, like women, can have multiple orgasms.

Prove It

Probably the most extensive laboratory investigation of male multiple orgasms was made by sex researchers William Hartman and

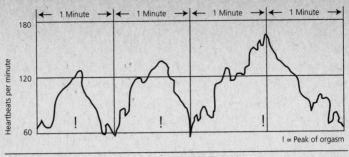

FIGURE 1. AROUSAL CHART FOR MULTI-ORGASMIC MAN   (Source: Hartman and Fithian)

Marilyn Fithian. They tested thirty-three men who claimed to be multi-orgasmic—that is, to be able to have two or more orgasms without losing their erection.

While these men had sex with their partners in the laboratory, Hartman and Fithian monitored their heart rates, which the researchers had chosen as the clearest method of identifying orgasms. At rest, the average heart rate is around 70 beats per minute; during orgasm it almost doubles, rising to about 120. After orgasm, the heart returns to its resting rate (see figure 1). They also measured pelvic contractions (most obvious in the involuntary squeezing of the anus), which coincided with the peaking of heart rate at orgasm. What they found was pretty surprising: the arousal charts for these men were identical to those of multi-orgasmic women.

Male and female sexuality may be more similar than is usually thought. Developmentally, this similarity makes sense, since male and female genitals come from the same fetal tissue. In their famous book *The G Spot and Other Recent Discoveries About Human Sexuality*, Alice Ladas, Beverly Whipple, and John Perry argued that male and female sexuality were almost identical. In addition to their much-reported discovery of the female "G spot" (which we will discuss more in chapter 4), they also suggested that men can experience multiple orgasms just like women.

During Hartman and Fithian's research, the average number of orgasms a multi-orgasmic man had was four. Some men had the minimum of two, and one had as many as sixteen! In a study by Marion Dunn and Jan Trost, most men reported having from two to nine orgasms per session.[3]

It is important to mention here that Taoist sexuality is not about numbers and keeping score, it is about satisfaction and cultivation. You can feel satisfied with one orgasm, with three orgasms, or with sixteen orgasms. You cultivate your sexuality as you deepen your awareness of your body's pleasure and increase your ability for intimacy with your partner. Each person and each sexual experience will be different, and the "right" number of orgasms will depend on your and your partner's desires at the time. When you become multi-orgasmic, you will never have to worry about how long you can last or how many orgasms your partner has, because you will both be able to have all the orgasms you could ever want.

The Little Death

As doctors, the Taoist masters were interested in sexuality as part of a larger concern for the health of the entire body. They practiced Sexual Kung Fu because they discovered that ejaculation drains a man's energy. You have probably also noticed this loss of energy and general feeling of fatigue after ejaculating. Even though you would like to be attentive to your partner's sexual and emotional needs, all your body wants to do is sleep. As one multi-orgasmic man put it, "Once I ejaculate, the pillow looks better than my girlfriend does."

The image of the unsatisfied woman whose lover ejaculates, grunts, and collapses on top of her is so common that it has become a cultural joke, but the exhaustion that men feel after ejaculating is as old as the first coital groan. Peng-Tze, a sex adviser to the famed Yellow Emperor, reported almost five thousand years ago: "After ejaculating, a man is tired, his ears buzz, his eyes are heavy, and he longs for sleep. He is thirsty and his limbs feel weak and stiff. In ejaculating he enjoys a brief moment of sensation but then suffers long hours of exhaustion."

Western folk wisdom agrees with the Taoists regarding the importance of conserving sexual energy. Athletes have long known the weakness and lethargy that follow ejaculation, abstaining from sex the night before the "big game." Artists have also felt the lingering effects on their work. Jazz musician Miles Davis explained in a *Playboy* magazine interview:

Davis: You can't come, then fight or play. You can't do it. When I get ready to come, I come. But I do not come and play.

Playboy: Explain that in layman's terms.

Davis: Ask Muhammad Ali. If he comes, he can't fight two minutes. Shit, he couldn't even whip me.

Playboy: Would you fight Muhammad Ali under those conditions, to prove your point?

Davis: You're goddamn right I'd fight him. But he's got to promise to fuck first. If he ain't going to fuck, I ain't going to fight. You give up all your energy when you come. I mean, *you give up all of it!* So, if you're going to fuck before a gig, how are you going to give something when it's time to hit?

Miles wasn't exactly a romantic, but he didn't mince words, either. As one of the world's greatest trumpet players, he knew how ejaculating decreased his stamina and depleted his art. Unfortunately, like most men, he didn't know that he could have had sex all he wanted, even have orgasmed, before any gig—as long as he didn't ejaculate. It might have even improved his "hitting."

Although the effects of ejaculating may be more obvious to professional musicians and prizefighters, all men eventually experience the same depletion from coming—which might more appropriately be called *going*. According to one multi-orgasmic man, "I really notice it in the morning if I ejaculate. I get up dragging my feet and I am tired by noon. When I have multiple orgasms without ejaculating, I wake up refreshed and I need less sleep." Another man who was recovering from a chronic illness explained: "My sexual desire has always been strong, so I ejaculated often, once or twice a day. And with every ejaculation my health got worse and worse because I was losing a lot of energy." Many men, especially young men, may not notice this feeling of depletion at first unless they ejaculate when they are sick or working hard.

In the West, we assume that ejaculation is an inevitable culmination of male arousal and the end of lovemaking. In China, however, doctors long ago saw what the French call *le petit mort*—"the little death" of ejaculation—as an avoidable betrayal of male pleasure and a dangerous depletion of male vitality.

DON JUANS, MONKS, AND MULTI-ORGASMIC WORMS

In a front-page story on December 3, 1992, the *New York Times* reported startling scientific research that seems to confirm the ancient Taoist insight about the toll that sperm production takes on a man's body. "These results are the last thing I had expected when I started doing the experiment," said Wayne Van Voorhies of the University of Arizona. "They were so startling that I did the work over four times to make sure I got it right. They basically say a lot of our preconceived notions [about male sexuality] just do not hold."[4]

Dr. Van Voorhies was studying simple but revealing worms called nematodes. What, you may ask, do worms have to do with your sexuality? Well, these nematodes are not just your everyday, garden-variety worms. "The genes and biochemical processes nematodes use," explains Dr. Philip Anderson of the University of Wisconsin, "are the same as those that humans and other mammals use." In scientific studies, nematodes are frequently used in place of human subjects.

Dr. Van Voorhies tested three kinds of male worms. The first group of worms was allowed to mate at will, which required frequent sperm production. On average, these Don Juan worms lived only 8.1 days. (Nematodes, in general, don't live very long.) The second group of worms was not allowed to mate at all. These, shall we say, *monastic* worms lived an average of 11.1 days. But even more startling, the third group, the *multi-orgasmic* worms that did not constantly have to produce sperm but were allowed to mate at will, lived close to 14 days—*over 50 percent longer* than the worms that needed to continually produce sperm!

The *Times* concluded: "The new work suggests that ceaseless sperm production takes its toll on a male, perhaps requiring the use of complex enzymes or biochemical processes that have harmful metabolic byproducts." The *Times* goes so far as to suggest that "the difference in life span between men and women just may be linked to sperm production. Women on average live about six years longer than men." There are other theories to explain the disparity in life expectancy between men and women, including differences in lifestyle and in hormones. Whether or not the production of sperm actually shortens your life, it certainly saps your strength.

Over two thousand years ago—long before experiments on nematodes—the Taoists described the importance of not ejaculating in the *Discourse on the Highest Tao Under Heaven*: "If a man has intercourse without spilling his seed, his vital essence is strengthened. If he does this twice, his hearing and vision are made clear. If three times, all his physical illness will disappear. The fourth time he will begin to feel inner peace. The fifth time his blood will circulate powerfully. The sixth time his genitals will gain new prowess. By the seventh his thighs and buttocks will become firm. The eighth time his body will radiate good health. The ninth time his life span will be increased." Ancient texts exaggerate to make their point, and it is unlikely that the above benefits occur in this exact order or at the exact specified time. However, it is clear that Taoists have long known the importance of conserving semen.

PROGENY AND PLEASURE

Looking at the simple arithmetic of sperm production helps explain the reason that ejaculation can be so taxing on your body. An average ejaculation contains 50 to 250 million sperm cells. (Theoretically speaking, if each sperm fertilized an egg, one to five ejaculations could repopulate the United States!) Every single one of those sperm cells is capable of creating half of an entire new human being. Any factory that produces 50 to 250 million products needs raw material, and in this case the raw material is you. Although your body produces a large amount of sperm each day, the value of this sperm should not be underrated. If your body does not need to replenish this sperm, according to the Tao, it is able to use this energy to strengthen your body and your mind. In the Taoist practice, this energy is used to improve your health, creativity, and spiritual growth.

Every time you ejaculate, your body assumes that it is getting ready to create a new life. According to the Tao, all of the organs and glands in your body give their best energy, what is called *orgasmic energy*. In many species, once this energy has been given, once the seed has been lost, the body of the animal starts to deteriorate. Salmon, for example, die soon after they spawn. Anyone who has spent time gardening knows that plants die or become dormant once they give their seed. Plants that are kept from going to seed live longer than those that are not. Though, luckily for us, we do not die after ejaculating, Taoists know that we are part of nature and that we must understand nature's laws.

According to *Sexual Behavior in the Human Male* (popularly known as the Kinsey Report), an average man ejaculates about five thousand times during his lifetime; some men ejaculate many, many more times. During the course of an average man's sex life (and this includes time spent locked in the bathroom), a man ejaculates 1 trillion sperm. Assuming that some of this ejaculation happens with a partner, the chances of his passing on his genetic code are pretty good. Most of the time, however, when we make love— not for progeny, but for pleasure—there is no need to spill our seed and deplete our bodies. So, if you make love only when you want to conceive a child, you will not need to practice Sexual Kung Fu. If, however, you want to have a multi-orgasmic and healthy sex life, read on.

CHAPTER TWO

Know Thyself

Exploring your body and understanding your arousal rate are essential to becoming multi-orgasmic. The best lovers are aware of both their own and their partner's desires. In chapter 4, we discuss how to satisfy your partner's desires, but first you must learn how to satisfy your own. In this chapter, we begin by briefly describing the basic facts about your sexual anatomy, your energy, your arousal, your ejaculation, and your orgasms. Then we offer some ideas for exploring your full potential for pleasure.

Your Body

PENIS

When most men think about their sexuality, they think about their penis. This is a logical place to start, since it is the most obvious part of our sexual anatomy. Strangely, there is still a lot of mystery and misinformation about this seemingly simple organ. To begin with, there are no bones or muscles in your penis. In fact, the penis is made primarily of spongy tissue. Because it has no muscle, you cannot enlarge it like your biceps—sorry. However, two or three inches of the penis is rooted inside the body in the pubococcygeus (pronounced *PEW-bo-cox-uh-GEE-us*) muscle—often just called the PC muscle—and it is possible, as we explain in the next chapter, to strengthen this muscle for stronger erections, stronger orgasms, and better ejaculatory control.

Since many men are concerned with the size of their penis and some are now even having penis-enlargement operations, we should take a moment to discuss the subject. Throughout human history, men have made many attempts to expand their so-called manhood—even the Taoists had their method, which we describe in chapter 8. But the truth is that the size of your erection is much less important than its strength and what you do with it. If you practice Sexual Kung Fu, you will have ample confirmation that you are "man enough" for any woman. If you are still concerned about the size of your penis, take a moment before running out to a plastic surgeon and read the section in chapter 8 called "Please, Sir, May I Have Some More: Enlarging Your Penis."

TESTICLES

Most men know that their sperm is produced in their testicles and may also know that normal body temperature is too hot for sperm production. (This is why tight underwear that keep your testicles close to your body can lower your sperm count.) Your testicles, however, are pulled into the body as they prepare to ejaculate. Pulling the testicles down away from the body, which we describe below, is one age-old technique for postponing ejaculation.

The vas deferens is a firm tube that extends from the testes to the prostate gland (see figure 2). Sperm move through this tube to the upper end, where they mix with secretions from the seminal vesicles and the prostate just before ejaculation. The secretions from the prostate constitute about one-third of your ejaculate and are responsible for its whitish color. The sperm are only a small part of the ejaculate, which is why a man who has had a vasectomy ejaculates about the same amount of fluid as he did before the operation.

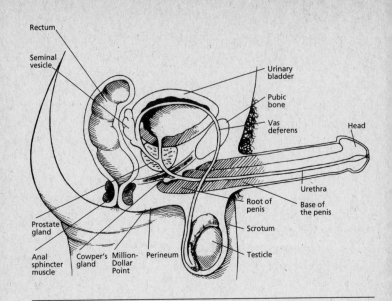

FIGURE 2. MAN'S SEXUAL ANATOMY

PROSTATE

The prostate is a gland that lies at the center of your pelvis, just behind the pubic bone, and just above the perineum (pronounced *pear-uh-NEE-um*). Most men have heard about the prostate only in connection with the dreaded and widespread prostate cancer, which occurs in approximately one in eleven American men. A healthy prostate is important for avoiding prostate cancer and for your long-term sexual well-being. You can help keep your prostate healthy and possibly reduce your risk of prostate cancer by doing the pelvic Sexual Kung Fu exercises suggested here and by massaging your prostate regularly. If you have prostate trouble or want to avoid having prostate trouble in the future, see the section called "My What? Preventing and Helping Prostate Problems" in chapter 8.

The prostate, like the G spot for women, is often highly sensitive to sexual stimulation. It has in fact been called "the male G spot." The authors of *The G Spot* concluded: "In men there is an orgasm triggered by the penis and one by the prostate." Men report that prostate orgasms are quite different from penile orgasms, emotionally as well physically. The authors of *The G Spot* suggest that this is equivalent to the difference women experience between clitoral and vaginal orgasms.

Like a woman's G spot, the prostate becomes increasingly sensitive to erotic stimulation as the man becomes aroused and approaches orgasm. This is why a prostate checkup at the doctor is quite different from prostate stimulation in bed with your lover. (You and your partner should remember that the body becomes engorged from front to back, so partners should wait until a man is highly aroused before attempting prostate stimulation.)

You can stimulate your prostate externally through your perineum at your Million-Dollar Point (more about this spot later in the chapter) or more directly through your anus. It is not always easy to reach by yourself if you are not very limber. Generally, the best position is lying on your back, either with your knees bent and your feet on the bed, or with your knees against your chest. In this position, you can insert a (well-lubricated) finger, curl it forward, and touch your prostate. You should feel something the size of a walnut an inch or two inside on the anterior (front) wall of your rectum. Gently rub the prostate back and forth. You can also thrust in and out at different speeds, which will also stimulate the highly sensitive nerves around your anus. If your partner is willing, she can do the same, but from a slightly easier angle. (Make sure your or your partner's nails are short.) If either you or your partner is not interested in venturing inside your anus, you can stimulate the anal sphincter and/or the perineum, which will also stimulate the prostate.

When prostate stimulation brings you to ejaculation, the fluid generally comes flowing out instead of spurting out. Keep in mind that this stimulation is very deep and very intense; as a result, it is even more difficult to control your arousal rate with prostate stimulation than it is with genital stimulation. So go slowly, and try not to push yourself over the edge.

PERINEUM

The perineum is an essential sexual landmark and was called "the Gate of Life and Death" by the Taoists. Its role in preventing ejaculation was a closely guarded secret. On the perineum just in front of the anus is the Million-Dollar Point, named to suggest its value to Sexual Kung Fu (see figure 2). This spot was originally called the Million-Gold-Piece Point (they didn't have dollars back in ancient China), because that is supposedly what it cost you to have a Taoist master teach you its exact location. (The ancient Taoist masters were holy men, but they also had to make a living.) In the next chapter, we discuss the role of the Million-Dollar Point in helping you control your ejaculation.

SEX MUSCLES

The pubococcygeus, or PC muscle, is a group of important pelvic muscles that run from your pubic bone ("pubo") in the front to your tailbone or coccyx ("coccygeus") in the back. These muscles form the basis of your sexual health and are essential for your becoming multi-orgasmic. In the following chapter we will describe exercises to strengthen these muscles.

If you have ever been forced to stay in bed for an extended period of time or to wear a cast, you know how your muscles atrophy and become weak when they are not used. This is equally true of your sex muscles. The penis actually withdraws into the body if it is not used regularly, as many older men who are not sexually active have witnessed. The Taoists knew that it is as important to exercise your sexual organs as any other part of your body.

ANUS

Its proximity to the prostate and its own high concentration of sensitive nerve endings make the anus a highly erogenous zone, as many men—both gay and straight—have discovered. Many people worry about the anus being "dirty" and consider it "unnatural" to stimulate the anus sexually. You should make sure that your anus is clean before you touch it and that you wash anything (such as a finger) that you use for anal stimulation before using it for vaginal stimulation to avoid spreading bacteria. Yet it is difficult to explain why the anus would be so sexually sensitive if stimulating it were "unnatural." Many heterosexual men also worry that they are gay or "will become gay" if they enjoy having their anuses stimulated, but there is no evidence to suggest a relationship between anal sensitivity and homosexuality. Homosexuality is a sexual orientation, not simply a sexual practice. Many gay men enjoy having their anuses stimulated, but many straight men do as well.

NIPPLES

Many men are surprised to find that their nipples are sensitive. Other men may require some regular stimulation to awaken their nerve endings. Nipple stimulation is one of the underrated and underexplored pleasures of male sexuality.

Your Energy

Understanding how the energy in your body works will allow you to expand genital orgasms into whole-body orgasms and to use your sexual energy to improve your creativity and health. As we mentioned in the introduction, Sexual Kung Fu developed as a branch of Chinese medicine. One of the world's oldest and most effective healing systems, Chinese medicine is responsible for the discovery of such successfully proven therapies as acupuncture and acupressure. According to Chinese medicine, in addition to the physical structures of your body, you also have physical energy that is constantly circulating through every cell of your body.

THE BODY ELECTRIC

As Western chemistry has become more refined, it is now able to demonstrate that our bodies are indeed filled with energy and electric charges. In the February 1984 issue of *Discover* magazine, K. C. Cole explained the comparison: "Electricity is almost certainly the most elusive of everyday things: It lives in the walls of our houses, and regulates the lives of our cells. . . . It runs electric trains and human brains. . . . Your entire body is a giant electric machine: body chemistry (like all chemistry) is based on electrical bonds."

Chinese medicine is based on a person's ability to maintain the proper circulation of this bioelectric energy through the body. If you have ever had acupuncture, you have experienced the circulation

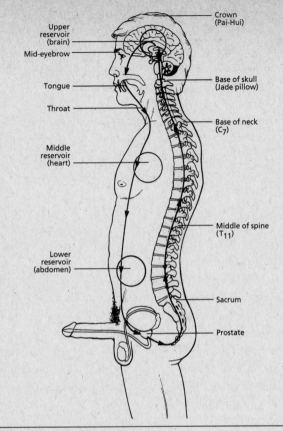

Upper reservoir (brain)

Mid-eyebrow

Tongue

Throat

Middle reservoir (heart)

Lower reservoir (abdomen)

Crown (Pai-Hui)

Base of skull (Jade pillow)

Base of neck (C_7)

Middle of spine (T_{11})

Sacrum

Prostate

FIGURE 3. THE MICROCOSMIC ORBIT

of this bioelectric energy, which the Chinese call *chi* (pronounced *CHEE*), in your own body. However, if you have not had this opportunity, there is a simple experiment you can do to feel your body's *chi*. Rub your hands together for ten seconds and then hold the palms about an inch apart. If you concentrate, you should be able to feel a flow of energy passing between them.

The idea of *chi* is not unique to China. Dr. John Mann and Larry Short, authors of *The Body of Light,* count forty-nine cultures around the world that have a word for *chi;* the words vary from *prana* in Sanskrit to *neyatoneyah* in Lakota Sioux to *num,* which means "boiling point," in the language of the Kalahari !Kung. The West is perhaps unique in its lack of an equivalent term. In the

West, we speak about feeling *energized* or having *low energy*, but with a few notable exceptions, we tend to ignore this important part of our physical body.

The concept of *chi* is gaining increasing acceptance in the medical establishment. A major transition occurred when President Richard Nixon reestablished diplomatic relations with China in 1972. In Beijing, Chinese doctors performed emergency surgery on *New York Times* correspondent James Reston, using only acupuncture for anesthesia. Since then many delegations of Western physicians to China have witnessed similar events.

Chi is just beginning to be understood in the terminology of Western science. Currently, several Western physicians are exploring the phenomenon, such as Robert Becker, a Syracuse University orthopedist and author of *The Body Electric*, who is trying to explain *chi* in relation to his work in bioelectricity and healing. It was Dr. Becker's research into electricity and its role in regenerating bones that led to the current method of using low-level electrical currents to stimulate the mending of fractures.

YOUR MICROCOSMIC ORBIT

You have bioelectric energy in every cell of your body. This energy also travels along certain well-defined circuits, called *meridians*, which acupuncture utilizes to regulate the amount of *chi* in any particular part of your body. The main circuit in the body is called the Microcosmic Orbit (see figure 3) and is made up of two channels, the Back Channel and the Front Channel (in Chinese medicine traditionally called the Governor Channel and the Functional Channel, respectively).

These channels are part of our earliest development. In utero, our body first resembles a flat disk. As the embryo develops, the disk folds over, leaving two seams, one along the midline of the back of our body and one along the front. The back seam can be seen in our spine, but the front line is more subtle. We rarely notice the front seam unless it does not close completely, as is the case with a child who is born with a harelip.

One multi-orgasmic man explained his understanding of the Microcosmic Orbit: "I think of the Microcosmic Orbit as a channel or meridian or route that has been discovered and tested over thousands of years to transform the raw biological energy used to create children into a lighter and more refined energy that can be used to improve one's health and one's lovemaking."

THE BACK CHANNEL

The Back Channel begins at the perineum and runs along the back of the body from the tip of the tailbone, up the spine and neck, to the crown of the head, and finally down the forehead to where it ends between the bottom of the nose and the upper lip, where there is an indentation.

THE FRONT CHANNEL

The Front Channel runs from the tip of your tongue to your throat and along the midline of your body down to your pubis and perineum. Touching your tongue to your palate closes the Microcosmic Orbit. The Front Channel is sometimes translated from the Chinese as the Conception Channel, and if you look very closely at the belly of a woman who is pregnant, you will generally see a dark line (which doctors call the *linea nigra*) that extends along part of this channel.

WHAT DOES ENERGY FEEL LIKE WHEN IT IS MOVING IN YOUR BODY? The fact is that you already have energy, or *chi,* moving through every part of your body. Without it, you would not be alive. Generally we just are not aware of this current of energy moving through our bodies. When we first become aware of *chi,* we may experience many different sensations. Some of the most common that people report are warmth, tingling, prickling (like the feeling of static electricity), pulsating, humming, bubbling, and buzzing. Some people feel it move slowly, while others feel a fast "rush." Though some people feel it move in a straight line along the Microcosmic Orbit, most people feel it more at some points along the orbit than at others.

HOW DOES *CHI* MOVE? There is a Taoist saying: "The mind moves and the *chi* follows." Wherever you focus your attention, the *chi* tends to gather and increase. As biofeedback experiments have now confirmed, focusing your attention on an area of the body can cause increased activity in the nerves and muscles in that area. The stronger the focus, the greater the movement of the *chi*. *Keep in mind that you are not pushing or pulling the* chi, *you are simply shifting your focus to another point.* Understanding this is crucial to developing an effective practice. However, you will not just be moving your attention over your skin, you will be experiencing a palpable flow of warm, tingling energy.

SEXUAL ENERGY

Sexual energy, or *ching-chi* (pronounced *JING-CHEE*) in Chinese, is one of the most obvious and powerful types of bioelectric energy. What we in the West call getting aroused, or getting horny, the Taoists thought of as the generating of sexual energy. Sexual Kung Fu practices are based on cultivating this sexual energy and using it to increase your overall energy and health. You must learn to draw your sexual energy out of your genitals and to circulate it through the rest of your body to truly master the Taoist techniques for experiencing multiple and whole-body orgasms and for improving your health.

As we mentioned in chapter 1, according to the Taoists all the parts of your body (including the brain, glands, organs, and senses) give their best energy during orgasm to create a new life. This is the power that goes into creating a child, but when procreation is not the goal, the Taoists believe, it is best to conserve this energy and channel it throughout your body for pleasure and health. *Since we are conceived through orgasm and orgasmic energy permeates every cell of our body, to stay healthy and active we need to feel this rejuvenating, orgasmic energy regularly—ideally, every day.*

Once you develop the ability to circulate sexual energy through your body, you will be able to feel this sensation throughout your body anywhere and at any time. Senior Healing Tao instructor Michael Winn explains: "Sexual energy is available to men twenty-four hours a day, but most men starve themselves because they believe they can satisfy themselves sexually only during a few minutes of intercourse. The most liberating thing for men is to discover that they have total access to and control over their sexual energy at any time."

You may be wondering whether all of this sexual energy will result in your feeling constantly aroused and in need of having sex, "an itch that needs to be scratched." On the contrary, men (and women) have sexual urges that need to be acted on or channeled in some way. In the West, we have tried to suppress or sublimate these desires, but according to the Tao this leads to physical and psychological imbalances.

When you practice self-cultivation, this feeling of arousal will result not in uncontrollable sexual urges but in an energetic, calm sense of well-being. One multi-orgasmic man explains the difference: "Before I started practicing Sexual Kung Fu, if I had not ejaculated in a while, my sexual urge would get stronger and stronger. I would look at pornography, look for one-night stands, or go to prostitutes. After ejaculating, this urge would disappear almost instantly and I couldn't understand why I had spent so much time and money trying to satisfy it. I would tell myself that I wouldn't do it next time, but I knew that after a while the sexual urge would return and I would do it all over again. When I finally started practicing Sexual Kung Fu, my sexual energy was still strong, but balanced. It was the first time in my life I was happy to be a man sexually, because I finally had control over my sexual energy."

As you practice, you may have more sexual energy than you are used to, and you will need to learn to channel this excess energy. As one multi-orgasmic man explained, "When I started the practice, all of my relationships became sexualized. I needed to learn to circulate and balance the energy." If this happens to you, the Cool Draw exercise described in the following chapter will help you transform this sexual energy into more neutral and less volatile physical energy, referred to earlier as *chi*. You can also take up Tai-chi or chi-kung (pronounced *CHEE-GUNG*) or other practices to help you ground and channel this additional energy. Exercise in general will help you to manage this additional energy.

Your Arousal

According to Taoism, we need to feel aroused, to feel the life-giving force of sexual energy, every day, because when we feel aroused, our bodies produce more sexual hormones, which in Taoism were considered the fountain of youth. (This need for arousal is why sex sells: we are drawn to images that stimulate this sexual energy and these sexual hormones.) When you learn how to circulate your sexual energy, you can feel this rejuvenating power at any time.

BECOMING AWARE OF YOUR AROUSAL

To learn to become multi-orgasmic, you will need to become increasingly aware of the speed at which you get aroused. This sounds pretty straightforward, but most men pay little attention to their arousal rate. Often men go from erection to ejaculation like race cars, without taking the time to notice, let alone enjoy, the sights along the way.

When you start to get sexually aroused, your penis increases in length and width as its spongy tissue fills with blood. As you become erect, valves close down in the veins, stopping the blood from returning to the body. Erection occurs spontaneously in newborn boys and in most men at least several times each night while dreaming.

Almost all men at some time in their lives experience the awkward situation in which they are unable to get an erection with a partner. The occasional inability to gain an erection may be caused by what psychologist Bernie Zilbergeld calls the "wisdom of the penis," telling you that there is something that needs to be addressed in your relationship, or it may simply be a sign that you are distracted by work or other pressures.

If a man repeatedly does not get an erection, he is called *impotent,* a word that also carries the suggestion of being weak and powerless. In Sexual Kung Fu, there is no such thing as "impotence," and by using the solo exercises to strengthen your erections and the Soft Entry technique in lovemaking, you should never have to worry about it again. If you are unable to get an erection when you want or if you want to know what to do when the situation arises (or doesn't), see "Snake Charming: Overcoming Impotence" in chapter 8.

THE STAGES OF ERECTION

Most men believe they are either horny or they're not, that they either have an erection or they don't. When we are young, we get erections so often and so quickly that it is hard to distinguish levels of arousal. The Taoists, however, noticed that there are actually four stages of erection—four *attainments,* as they called them.

The first is *firmness* (also referred to as *lengthening*).
The second is *swelling*.
The third is *hardness*.
The fourth is *heat*.

Your erection is not then just a static appendage, but undergoes a process that reflects your level of arousal. Western physicians have recently confirmed these four stages of erection, although describing them in somewhat more technical terms.[1]

Healing Tao instructor Walter Beckley described the four stages like this: "In the first stage, your penis starts to *move and become erect.* In the second stage, it's *firm, but not hard*—not really hard enough to penetrate (unless you use the Soft Entry technique). In the third stage, it is *erect and hard.* In the fourth stage, it is *stiff and really hot.* This last stage is also when your testicles draw into your body. It is much easier to avoid ejaculating when you can remain in the erect and hard third stage. Pulling the sexual energy up helps keep the penis from getting to the final, stiff and hot stage. Relaxing is also essential, as is trying to be aware of when you move into that anxious, explosive fourth stage when ejaculation is imminent."

THE SECRET OF MALE SEXUALITY

As we mature as lovers, we are able to gain some control of our arousal in an attempt to please our partners. Generally called our *staying power,* this ability is often achieved by learning to distract ourselves from our arousal (thinking about baseball statistics, for example) rather than by learning to sensitize ourselves to it. True ejaculatory control comes from knowing your individual arousal rate, not ignoring it. As you learn to feel your rising pleasure more, it will become easier for you to take the multi-orgasmic path.

BUT ISN'T SEX SUPPOSED TO BE ABOUT RELAXING AND LETTING GO? To experience sexual pleasure, men must certainly relax and let go, but if we relax and let go too much, we ejaculate and then most, if not all, of the pleasure is gone. Knowing when to let go of our sexuality and when to control it is the essence of Sexual Kung Fu, and the secret to male sexuality.

Your Ejaculation

The ejection of semen from your body actually occurs in two parts. In the *contractile* (sometimes called "emission") phase, the prostate contracts and empties semen into the urethra. In the *expulsion* phase, the semen is propelled down the urethra and out the penis. When you become multi-orgasmic you will experience the pleasurable pelvic contractions—what we will call *contractile-phase orgasm*, which is felt as a popping or fluttering sensation in your prostate—without actually ejaculating. Though some men have multiple *ejaculations* during one love-making session (this is easiest for teenage boys), it should be clear by now that this is quite different from multiple—*non*ejaculatory—orgasms.

As you are becoming highly aroused, a few drops of clear fluid may trickle out of your penis. This preseminal fluid comes from the prostate and other glands, such as the Cowper's glands, which produce an alkaline fluid used to lubricate the urethra and pave the way for the sperm. The Taoists called this liquid *water*, which they distinguished from *milk*, or semen. This fluid is perfectly natural and signals the approach of contractile-phase orgasm. It may, however, have a number of sperm in it. This is the "pre-ejaculate" that they warn you about in sex-education classes, so you will need to make sure that you continue to use birth control even if you don't ejaculate. However, if you have nonejaculatory orgasms, the chances of you and your partner having an unplanned pregnancy are much lower.

WHERE DOES THE SEMEN GO WHEN I DON'T EJACULATE? The semen is broken down and reabsorbed by the body, just as the sperm are reabsorbed in a man who has had a vasectomy. However, the effects of the Taoist techniques on the body are very different from those of a vasectomy. With a vasectomy, the vas deferens is cut just above the testicles and the sperm have nowhere to go. They are eventually reabsorbed, but many men complain about feeling congestion in the testicles and pelvis. If you have had a vasectomy, it is additionally important for you to practice the Testicle

Massage exercise (see chapter 8) and to circulate your sexual energy.[2] Both of these techniques help the body absorb the sperm and relieve any feeling of fullness or congestion. The involuntary contractions of the contractile-phase orgasms that you will learn to experience without ejaculation also massage the prostate, which helps to relieve congestion and keep the prostate healthy.

CAN NOT EJACULATING HURT ME? The Taoists have been practicing the techniques given in this book for thousands of years without negative side effects, and in fact with great improvement to their health and longevity. From their study of multi-orgasmic men in the West, Dunn and Trost concur: "None of our subjects has yet developed erectile or ejaculatory difficulties. Our older multiple orgasmic men maintain firm erections after one or more orgasms. In our clinical experience we have not seen men who become sexually dysfunctional following experimentation with multiple orgasms."

FINDING THE WAY

Where Did It Go?

I didn't ejaculate, but I lost my erection. What happened?
There is one other thing that can happen to your semen besides its being ejaculated or reabsorbed by your body. Occasionally, as you are practicing the Taoist techniques, you may experience an orgasm without ejaculating but lose your erection. If this is not simply due to a decrease in your arousal, you probably have experienced a *retrograde*, or backward, ejaculation. When this occurs, the semen goes into your bladder and passes harmlessly out of your body the next time you urinate. Since you lose your erection and eventually your sperm (when you urinate), you have not done the practice correctly, but you should also know that you have not done yourself any harm.[3] Hartman and Fithian explain: "What's important to know is that there is

no apparent harm to the body when a retrograde ejaculation takes place. All that happens is that if the ejaculation is complete the penis becomes flaccid, as it usually does after ordinary ejaculations." If you lose your erection and are curious, you can urinate into a cup. If it's cloudy, you had a retrograde ejaculation. You may not want to do this urine test except when you are practicing by yourself, since it might seem a bit clinical during a candlelit night of lovemaking.

Your Orgasm

The male orgasm lies on the precipice of ejaculation. If you rush forward to experience it, you will fall over the edge and down into the ravine of postejaculatory stupor. Though many men continue to feel pleasure after they have ejaculated, most find themselves at the bottom of their arousal slope, having to climb slowly back up. The five to ten strong ejaculatory contractions are quite pleasurable; otherwise, most men would not see them as the goal of their desire. Ejaculatory orgasm may seem like a thrilling ride, but after you experience the prolonged and ecstatic sexual aerobatics of multiple orgasms, this ejaculatory descent will seem pretty tame and, by comparison, pretty disappointing. "After I have a 'squirt' orgasm," as one multi-orgasmic man described ejaculation, "I feel like I've been on a six-second roller coaster—after standing in line for two hours!"

HOW CAN I EXPERIENCE MULTIPLE ORGASMS?   As with any orgasm you have had, you begin by getting sexually aroused, whether from a thought, the sight of your lover, your lover's voice, or your lover's touch. (In the case of adolescent boys, the blowing of the wind can suffice.) This arousal generally leads to an erection, and with increasing stimulation you pass through an excitement phase until you reach your *contractile phase*. The contractile phase is a crucial fork in the road, one direction leading to ejaculation and the other to multiple orgasms (see figure 4).

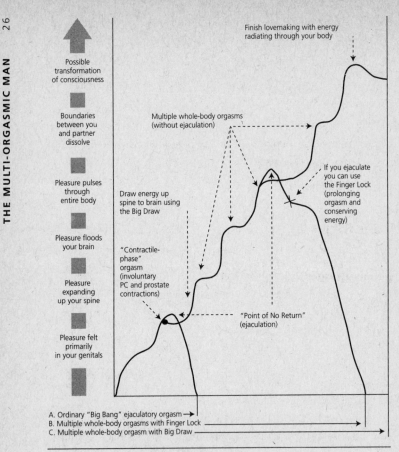

Possible transformation of consciousness

Boundaries between you and partner dissolve

Pleasure pulses through entire body

Pleasure floods your brain

Pleasure expanding up your spine

Pleasure felt primarily in your genitals

Finish lovemaking with energy radiating through your body

Multiple whole-body orgasms (without ejaculation)

Draw energy up spine to brain using the Big Draw

If you ejaculate you can use the Finger Lock (prolonging orgasm and conserving energy)

"Contractile-phase" orgasm (involuntary PC and prostate contractions)

"Point of No Return" (ejaculation)

A. Ordinary "Big Bang" ejaculatory orgasm →
B. Multiple whole-body orgasms with Finger Lock
C. Multiple whole-body orgasm with Big Draw

FIGURE 4. YOUR ORGASMIC POTENTIAL
Instead of the ordinary "Big Bang" ejaculatory orgasm (A), with Sexual Kung Fu you can draw your sexual energy up during your contractile phase (before ejaculation) and have multiple whole-body orgasms. If you ejaculate, you can use the Finger Lock, which will prolong your orgasm and conserve energy (B). If you avoid ejaculation, you can use the Big Draw to finish lovemaking with energy radiating through your body (C).

During the contractile phase, you will feel a series of prostate contractions lasting three to five seconds. These pleasurable pelvic orgasms are what we have been calling *contractile-phase orgasms*. Though the intensity of these orgasms varies and they can often be as intense as regular ejaculatory orgasms, at first they may be quite mild. Now is the moment of truth. Instead of continuing to the point of no return, past which you must ejaculate, you will stop or otherwise decrease your stimulation momentarily—long enough for you to gain control of your arousal rate.

You can also squeeze your PC muscle around your fluttering prostate, which will help you maintain some control over these spasms. Drawing the energy away from your genitals and up your spine as we describe in the next chapter will help relieve the pressure and the urge to ejaculate. Your level of excitement will decrease slightly in preparation for another genital orgasm. With multiple orgasms, your arousal is like a wave that rises to a peak and then, instead of cresting over and crashing, is swept up by a larger wave and on to an even higher peak.

One important point: if you strive for contractile-phase orgasms, there is a good chance you will crest over into ejaculation. Most men find that they must stop their arousal just before reaching contractile-phase orgasm and let themselves relax into it. Many multi-orgasmic men describe themselves as mentally falling *backward* into nonejaculatory orgasms instead of falling *forward* into ejaculation. The idea is to stay as close as possible to the point of ejaculatory inevitability—reveling in the contractile-phase orgasm—without cresting over into ejaculation. You will feel the pleasure and release of the prostate contractions, the PC contractions, and the anal-sphincter contractions.

How close together you experience these multiple contractile-phase orgasms depends on you. You will experience waves of satisfying pleasure, which, if your partner is multi-orgasmic, will help you harmonize your sexual desire. You will not have to worry about giving your partner "her orgasm(s)" and then getting "your orgasm." Rather, you both have the potential for multiple peaks of orgasmic pleasure.

FINDING THE WAY

Oops!

If you are having difficulty separating your orgasm from your ejaculation, you can begin drawing the sexual energy up your spine before you orgasm. According to the Tao, the real key to whole-body pleasure and healing is the circulation of this sexual energy through the Microcosmic Orbit. Once you start drawing sexual energy up, you may discover that you have "orgasmic" feelings in your brain or in other parts of your body or in your entire body.

Voluntarily squeezing your PC muscle around your prostate will also help you develop sensitivity in your pelvis and control the contractile-phase orgasms that cause your prostate to contract in pleasurable involuntary spasms.

When you do crest over into ejaculation, which you will do many times while you are learning—and even occasionally afterward—don't get frustrated or disappointed. Enjoy the pleasurable contractions of your penis that accompany ejaculation and realize that there is always another opportunity to experience more peaks later. Remember, the practice takes time and intimacy, with yourself and with your partner.

WHAT IS THE DIFFERENCE BETWEEN MULTIPLE ORGASMS AND *WHOLE-BODY* MULTIPLE ORGASMS? Each genital orgasm helps release the tension that results from the built-up sexual energy and the increased flow of blood into your pelvis. Several pelvic—nonejaculatory—orgasms are extremely satisfying (and energizing), but as you develop your orgasmic capacity, you will no doubt want to expand these pelvic orgasms throughout the rest of your body, which is the real secret of the Tao.

Whole-body multiple orgasms also begin with the contractile-phase release of pelvic orgasms, but instead of keeping the sexual energy (and the pleasure) in your pelvis, you draw your sexual energy up your spine, into your brain, and throughout your entire body, as we will show you step by step in the next chapter.

Most men do not even realize they can reach these sexual peaks. Not only do they experience only one orgasm (which, for them, is the same as ejaculation), but they experience this orgasm almost exclusively in their genitals. In *Everything You Always Wanted to Know About Sex (But Were Afraid to Ask)*, Dr. David Reuben describes orgasm as it is typically understood by Western sexologists: "For orgasm to occur, the full force of the body's entire nervous system must be concentrated on the sexual organs. Successful orgasm requires that every microvolt of electrical energy be mobilized and directed toward the penis and clitoris-vagina." Reuben, however, goes no further than a discussion of what the Taoists knew was just the first level of orgasm, or *genital orgasm*.

As represented in the illustration of your orgasmic potential (see figure 4), you can learn not only to experience multiple orgasms, but also to expand your orgasms from your genitals to your brain to your entire body. In the words of one multi-orgasmic man, "A whole-body orgasm is unbelievable. Once you experience it you never go back to a genital orgasm."

WHAT EXACTLY DO WHOLE-BODY ORGASMS FEEL LIKE? Everyone experiences this orgasmic high slightly differently, which makes it difficult to describe in general terms. The experience is often so intense that people resort to mystical language (using phrases like "oneness with the universe") that is difficult to understand if you have not experienced what is being described. However, people frequently have more concrete sensations such as warmth, tingling, vibrating, or pulsating throughout their body. The best way to know what you might feel is through the descriptions of men who have had whole-body multiple orgasms.

One multi-orgasmic man described his first experience of a whole-body orgasm: "We were making love and I thought I was going to come and I started doing my deep breathing, and as I was doing my deep breathing my head started to kind of electrify—to tingle. Like little sparks going on inside, tingly little things that went up the back of my neck a little bit. It started rushing back and forth in my head. And I almost thought I was going to get dizzy—it was *so good*. And I thought, 'If this goes any further, I might just lift off!' It lasted for—it's hard to know what time is like in bed—but at least a minute. It was a *long* orgasm. Just tingling, tingling, tingling. It would go away and then come back. My body was ringing like a bell."

Another man described his first experience of a multiple orgasm like this: "It was not localized in my genitals. My whole body started vibrating. And I thought, 'Well, I don't know what is going on here.' And so at first I was a little alarmed, but it felt good, so I just relaxed and let it happen."

Another multi-orgasmic man described his experience this way: "My growing sexual arousal is less active, less hot, less wild than an ejaculatory orgasm. It is more balanced and controlled. As the pleasure and pressure build up, they can flow into the Microcosmic Orbit and through my whole body. The goal is not to shoot the sperm, but to feel this vibrating energy throughout my whole body, to activate love and tenderness, and to expand my spirit. The whole body is much more relaxed, especially at the moment of orgasm."

Finally, one multi-orgasmic man compared the experience to an ejaculatory orgasm like this: "The feeling of the whole-body orgasm is more subtle, complete, satisfying. The whole process is not a feeling of a short explosion but of a longer and slower implosion. I don't feel empty afterward, which is easy to understand because with an explosion something leaves your body, but with an implosion you still have it in you. There remains a deep satisfaction on the physical, emotional, and spiritual levels, which stays sometimes for hours, sometimes for days."

In the West, we have limited our definition of an orgasm to pulsations that take place in our pelvis (prostate) and genitals (penis), but the ancient Taoists understood that an orgasm is any pulsation (contraction and expansion) and can take place in any part of your body. Michael Winn explains: "You can have an orgasmic pulsation in the whole body or in any part of the body. One of your organs can have an orgasm. Your brain can have an orgasm. You wouldn't know you are having an orgasm in your penis or in your prostate unless your brain was having an orgasm, too."

DISCRETE AND CONTINUOUS MULTIPLE ORGASMS

It is important to point out that whole-body orgasms are so intense that it is often hard to know where one ends and another begins. The waves of pleasure that you experience make any attempt to "keep score" truly irrelevant. Hartman and Fithian's laboratory research (see chapter 1) suggests that men (and women) can in fact have both *discrete* (separate) multiple orgasms and *continuous* multiple orgasms.

With discrete multiple orgasms, you have a peak orgasmic experience and then the orgasm subsides, but it is then followed by another discrete orgasm. With continuous multiple orgasms, you have a peak orgasmic experience that may grow more or less intense, but you never leave the orgasmic state entirely. Hartman and Fithian recorded these two different types of orgasms by looking at heart rate, which in discrete multiple orgasms would return to its baseline figure (around seventy beats per minute) between orgasms. In continuous multiple orgasms the heart rate reached a number of peaks without returning to the baseline in between (see figure 19, page 98). Finally, these discrete and continuous orgasms can combine to make countless combinations of pleasurable peaks. The possibilities are really endless. It's a far cry from the six-second orgasm most men have learned to settle for as the "normal" male orgasm.

SEX AND SPIRITUALITY

If you are practicing the duo practice (that is, with a partner), you may also feel your sexual energy circulate through her and her sexual energy circulate through you. Eventually you may feel as if the physical boundaries between the two of you dissolve. Many men have experienced this oneness with a partner, or even a feeling of oneness with the universe, during extraordinarily intimate lovemaking. With Sexual Kung Fu, you will learn how to return to this place regularly with your partner and even by yourself. This kind of sexual union with another person and between yourself and the universe can actually result in a transformation of consciousness. It is for this reason that sexuality in the East has often been seen as part of the spiritual path, and not as something opposed to it. (We discuss the connection between sexuality and spirituality more in chapter 5, in the section called "Sexing the Spirit.")

CHAPTER THREE

Becoming a Multi-Orgasmic Man

Now that you have a better understanding of your sexuality and its true potential, it is time to become multi-orgasmic. This ability requires developing both your sexual strength and your sexual sensitivity. As mentioned in the introduction, most men who practice the exercises in this chapter will begin to experience multiple orgasms within a week or two and will master the technique within three to six months. Some with strong sexual energy and sexual sensitivity may experience them the first time they try, while others with weaker energy or less sensitivity may take longer than six months to become regularly multi-orgasmic. It also depends on your dedication to the practice. We give you these time frames as an estimate, but the most important thing is not to get discouraged. If you persevere, you will get it.

Breathing Basics

Strange as it may seem, learning to control your ejaculation and to become multiply orgasmic begins with strengthening and deepening your breathing. As is true in all martial arts and meditative practices, your breath is the gate through which you can gain control of your body. Breathing is both involuntary *and* voluntary. In other words, we breathe regularly without thinking about it, but we can also choose to change the rhythm or depth of our breathing. This use of the mind to cultivate the body is the very basis of Sexual Kung Fu.

Your breathing is also related to your heart rate. If you are breathing quickly and shallowly, as after running, your heart rate increases. If you are breathing slowly and deeply, your heart rate decreases. As we learned earlier, increased heart rate is part of orgasm and breathing quickly is one sign of orgasm's approach. So the first step in controlling your arousal rate, and therefore your ejaculation, is deep and slow breathing.

BELLY BREATHING

Most of us breathe very shallowly, generally into our chest and shoulders, which allows only a small amount of oxygen to be absorbed by our lungs. Belly breathing—breathing deeply into the bottom of our lungs—is the way a newborn child breathes. If you watch a sleeping newborn, you will see the child's entire belly rise and fall with each breath. Belly breathing allows us to replace stagnant air at the bottom of our lungs with fresh, oxygen-filled air. This is the healthiest way to breathe, but we lose this natural ability as stress and anxiety cause us to cut our breathing short. This anxious breathing is confined to our upper chest. When we are happy and laughing, we are able once again to breathe into our belly. In this exercise, you will learn to belly breathe as you did when you were young.

FINDING THE WAY

Inhale Through Your Nose

When practicing any of the exercises in this book, always inhale through your nose, which filters and warms the air. When you inhale through your mouth, you breathe unfiltered, unwarmed air, which is harder for your body to assimilate.

BELLY BREATHING

1. Sit on a chair with your back straight and your feet touching the floor about shoulder width apart.

2. Place your hands over your navel and relax your shoulders.

3. Inhale through your nose and feel your lower abdomen expand at the navel area (below and around it) so that it bulges outward. Your diaphragm will also descend (see figure 5).

4. Keeping your chest relaxed, exhale with some force to pull the lower abdomen back in, as if you were pulling your navel back toward your spine. Also feel your penis and testicles pull up.

5. Repeat steps 3 and 4 eighteen to thirty-six times.

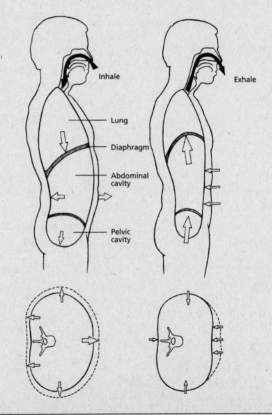

FIGURE 5. BELLY BREATHING

A few minutes of belly breathing each day will teach your body to breathe deeply on its own, even when you are asleep. When you are in the heat of passion, this ability to control your breathing will be essential to stopping yourself from ejaculating and to expanding the feeling of orgasm throughout your whole body.

Once you learn not to ejaculate, it is very important to do this deep-breathing exercise or eventually just to breathe deeply on your own. It will help circulate your sexual energy through your body and absorb it into your organs. Belly breathing also massages the organs and prostate and can relieve the full feeling many men experience when they first stop ejaculating.

Although it is not as important to exhale through your nose as it is to inhale, it is still preferable. Some people, however, find it easier to exhale through their mouth when breathing deeply. See what works best for you.

FINDING THE WAY

Belly Laughing

If you are having a hard time with belly breathing, as many Westerners do, you can practice belly *laughing* instead. A belly laugh is the kind of laugh that makes your whole abdomen shake. It is not the fake salesman's laugh; it is the genuine laugh you have with your close friends. It is the kind of laugh that can make your stomach ache, since most of us do not use these muscles very often.

To belly laugh, sit in a chair with your back straight and your feet on the floor about shoulder width apart. Place your hands over your belly and start to laugh (from your belly). Feel your stomach vibrate. This belly laughing will help relax your diaphragm and let you breathe from your belly. It also will help you generate a lot of energy, which you will later learn to circulate through your body for better orgasms and better health.

EXERCISE 2

CENTURY COUNT

1. Slowly inhale (expanding your belly) and exhale (flattening your belly). Count each complete inhalation and exhalation as one breath.

2. Continue breathing from the belly and counting from one to one hundred, thinking only about your breathing.

3. If you notice that your mind has strayed, start again.

4. Practice this exercise twice a day until you can count to one hundred with ease.

Increasing Your Concentration

This exercise builds on the belly breathing you just learned and will help you improve your concentration. In this exercise you count one hundred breaths without letting your mind wander. (A complete inhalation and exhalation is one breath.) This is very simple, but not easy. Most people have difficulty counting to ten, let alone one hundred, without letting their mind wander. One multi-orgasmic man explained his practice: "I go to the gym and I'll sit in the sauna and count my breath in and out as one, in and out as two, all the way to one hundred. Sometimes I'll be breathing and counting, and suddenly around fifty or sixty I realize I'm thinking about stocks or something and I can't remember what number I'm at, so I go back to one and I just start counting again until I get to one hundred."

Strengthening Your Sex Muscles

Now it is time to develop your sexual strength. The pubococcygeus muscle, or PC muscle, which we mentioned in the last chapter, is the muscular sling that stretches from the pubic bone in the front to the tailbone in the back (see figure 6). Most men feel their PC muscle at their perineum, just behind their testicles and in front of their anus. This is the muscle you use to stop yourself from urinating when you can't find a toilet. The PC muscle is also responsible

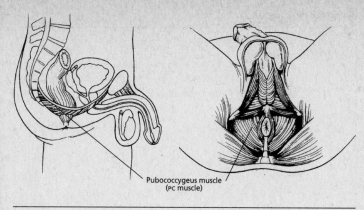

Pubococcygeus muscle
(PC muscle)

FIGURE 6. THE PC MUSCLE

for the rhythmic contractions in your pelvis and anus during orgasm. In *The G Spot,* Ladas, Whipple, and Perry describe the importance of the PC muscle: "If men increase the strength of their pubococcygeus muscle, they too can learn to become multiply orgasmic and separate between orgasm and ejaculation." Your orgasm builds from your prostate, so learning how to squeeze on the prostate with your pelvic muscles is essential. In addition to having more and better orgasms, you will by this squeezing prevent hardening and swelling of the prostate and help avoid or heal prostate problems.

The PC muscle (which surrounds the prostate gland) serves as a valve around the genitals that you will learn to open and close. You can feel this muscle working when you are trying to push out those last few drops of urine. Women feel it most when they are trying to push out a baby. Women who have developed strong PC muscles can hold a man's penis in their vagina more tightly, increasing sensation for both partners.

The PC muscle is also what allows animals to wag their tails. Strangely, the word *penis* literally means "tail" in Latin. So what you are going to do with these exercises is learn to "wag your tail" to strengthen your erections, intensify your orgasms, and separate your orgasms from ejaculation.

EXERCISE 3

STOPPING THE STREAM

1. When you are about to urinate, stand on your toes and the balls of your feet. If necessary, you can use the wall for support.

2. Inhale deeply.

3. Exhale slowly, forcefully push out the urine while pulling up on your perineum and clenching your teeth.

4. Inhale and contract your PC muscle to stop the flow of urine midstream.

5. Exhale and start urinating again.

6. Repeat steps 4 and 5 three to six times or until you have finished urinating.

STOPPING THE STREAM

The easiest way to find your PC muscle is to stop the flow of urine by clamping down the muscles in your pelvis the next time you are going to the bathroom. Stopping yourself from peeing was one of the first acts of control you learned to have over your body. Using your ability to control your urine flow can now help you control your ejaculation, because the urinary duct, the ejaculatory duct, and the seminal-vesicle duct all pass through the prostate. (This is why when a man's prostate is enlarged, he has problems urinating and ejaculating.)

FINDING THE WAY

Emptying Your Bladder

Because the bladder and the prostate are so close, you should also urinate before self-pleasuring or lovemaking whenever your bladder feels full. A full bladder will make you feel like you need to ejaculate and can actually make it more difficult for you to stop yourself from ejaculating.

If you have a strong PC muscle, you should be able to stop the flow of urine midstream and then start it again. If this is difficult for you, your PC muscle is weak. Stopping the flow of urine may sting at first. This is perfectly normal and should stop within a few weeks, unless for some reason you have an infection, in which case you should wait until you have seen a doctor and cleared it up before continuing with the practice. If your muscle becomes sore, you just need practice. Pulling up on your perineum as you push out the urine will help you urinate with more force and will help strengthen your kidneys, prostate gland, and bladder in addition to your PC muscle.

Although standing on your toes and clenching your teeth will help intensify your practice, *the most important part of the practice is simply to stop and start urinating as many times as you can.* One multi-orgasmic man described his "peeing practice" this way: "Whenever I go to the bathroom now, I try to stop and go at least three times. And if I am in a fun mood and I am not in a rush, I will try to just stop, go, stop, go, sometimes maybe five or six or seven times."

PC PULL-UPS

The importance of the PC muscle was discovered in the West during the 1940s by Arnold Kegel, a gynecologist. He developed the famous Kegel (pronounced *KAY-gul*) exercises, which help many pregnant women control their bladders and which can ease childbirth. Women found that these exercises could also increase their sexual desire, intensify their orgasms, and help them become multi-orgasmic. Strengthening this muscle, as we have mentioned earlier, is equally important for a man's pelvic health and sexual pleasure.

There are many different exercises for strengthening your PC muscle that have been taught in the West, most of them adaptations of Kegel's original technique. All of them teach you to contract and relax the muscle, although the number of repetitions and the amount of time suggested for holding the contractions vary. The following exercise is based on the Taoist awareness that the

EXERCISE 4

PC PULL-UPS

1. Inhale and concentrate on your prostate, perineum, and anus.

2. As you exhale, contract your PC muscle around your prostate and around your anus while at the same time contracting the muscles around your eyes and mouth.

3. Inhale and relax, releasing your PC, eye, and mouth muscles.

4. Repeat steps 2 and 3, contracting your muscles as you exhale and releasing them as you inhale, nine to thirty-six times.

circular muscles of the body (including the muscles around the eyes, mouth, perineum, and anus) are connected. By squeezing the muscles around your eyes and mouth, you can increase the force of your PC Pull-Ups. It is easiest to begin practicing this exercise while sitting, but later on you can do this exercise while standing or lying down.

Although contracting your eyes and your lips will help you squeeze your PC muscle around your prostate and anus, *the most important part of the practice is simply contracting and releasing your PC muscle as often as you can*, which you can do practically any-where—while driving, while watching TV, while sending a fax, while in a boring meeting. You can see how many contractions you can do during a red light, or you can hold a single contraction until the light turns green.

Try to do the exercise at least two or three times a day, although you can do it as many times as you like. Your muscles may get sore, just as they do after doing regular pull-ups. Don't push yourself too far; increase the number and frequency gradually. Consistency is more important than quantity. One way to help develop a daily routine is to connect your practice to daily events, like getting up in the morning, taking a shower, or lying in bed at night.

According to the authors of *The G Spot*, a man with a healthy PC muscle should be able to raise and lower a towel on his erect penis by contracting this muscle. (In the more advanced Taoist practice, you can even learn to use weights to strengthen your pelvic muscles.) For now, you may want to try raising and lowering a towel, but you probably should avoid having an audience. As the authors of *The G Spot* correctly point out, "'performance anxiety' is the archenemy of male erection."

Self-Pleasuring and Self-Cultivation

Next, you need to cultivate your sexual sensitivity. The easiest way to develop this awareness is through self-pleasuring. Unfortunately, most of us in the West did not grow up with an understanding of sex and sexual energy as natural and essential parts of our overall health. From the first time you started touching your "privates," your parents may have subtly, or not so subtly, told you to keep your hands out of your pants. Though this probably did not stop you from locking yourself in your bedroom or in the bathroom, you probably have some guilt and embarrassment about masturbating. You are not alone.

Christianity's ambivalence toward sex, especially sex that is not procreative, still influences Western society and sexual mores. For example, in 1994 Dr. Joycelyn Elders, the U.S. surgeon general, was forced to resign for stating publicly that masturbation "is a part of human sexuality." Therefore, it is worth mentioning that Christianity's prohibition of masturbation, which at one time was called *onanism,* is based on a misreading of the biblical story of Onan. Onan was punished for refusing to impregnate the wife of his dead brother, as was the custom at the time. His "sin" had nothing to do with masturbation.[1]

PLAYING WITH YOURSELF

Taoist sexuality was developed as a branch of medicine, not morality.[2] It therefore does not prohibit any form of human sexual activity but simply tries to teach people how to stay healthy while engaging in it. The Taoist masters saw masturbation, which they called *solo cultivation* or *genital exercise,* as an essential way of developing ejaculatory control and of learning to circulate sexual energy to revitalize the body. (Remember, solo cultivation, which we will refer to as both *self-cultivation* and *self-pleasuring,* does not include ejaculation.)

According to the Tao, play is one of the best ways to learn, and "playing with ourselves" is an excellent way to strengthen our genitals and our sexual energy. Many people worry about masturbating "too much," but the Taoists knew that there is no such thing—as long as one learns to control ejaculation. Too much ejaculation is the problem: it drains men of their strength, but this can happen with intercourse as well as self-pleasuring.

According to Kinsey and more recent surveys, almost all boys— and most men—masturbate.[3] Prohibiting or discouraging a natural part of child sexuality turns boys into sexual thieves, forcing them to steal their pleasure. It is quite possible that most men ejaculate so quickly because they grew up trying to "get off" before they "got caught." Dr. Wardell Pomeroy, in his book *Boys and Sex,* explains that since almost all boys masturbate, they should learn to do so slowly and for extended periods of time so that they will be able to make love longer when they eventually become sexually active.

The Taoists would add that boys should learn to pleasure themselves without ejaculating. Young boys or teenagers who ejaculate too much can find that their energy and motivation for other activities decreases significantly. When one of the authors of this book, Mantak Chia, was growing up in Thailand, he sat next to a boy in school who had repeated the fourth grade four times. The boy masturbated each day in class four or five times and ejaculated into a bottle. Obviously, his was an extreme case, but according to Taoism, his failure in school was quite understandable. He was literally draining himself and his brain. The expression "screwing your brains out" is an accurate description of the stupor that occurs after repeated ejaculation.

Many men (and women) who are married or in relationships continue to pleasure themselves. In 1972, the American Medical Association advised physicians in a book entitled *Human Sexuality,* "Masturbation is practiced by men and women of all ages, often as a supplement to marital coitus, and women tend to masturbate more as they grow older." (Estimates suggest that about 70 percent of married men—and married women—pleasure themselves.⁴) Self-pleasuring does not take the place of sex with a partner, but it can serve as a valuable complement. A recent national sex study sponsored by the University of Chicago found that people who are having sex regularly with a partner actually pleasure themselves *more* than people who are not.⁵

Pleasuring yourself can help relieve built-up tension when you need a sexual release more than intimacy. It also can help when your partner is tired, distracted, or does not have the same sexual appetite. (If your partner generally has a lower sex drive, make sure to recommend that she read chapter 6 and that you both read the section called "The Seasons of Our Sex Lives" in chapter 9.) If for whatever reason you feel that you just can't pleasure yourself, you can learn to become multi-orgasmic with your partner instead. It may take a little longer, that's all. You can also do the exercises you have already learned: Belly Breathing, Century Count, Stopping the Stream, and PC Pull-Ups.

Pleasuring ourselves is not something we are taught to do. Considering the outcry that occurred when Surgeon General Elders suggested that masturbation "perhaps should be taught," it is unlikely that it will be introduced into the curriculum anytime soon. Most of us learn how to masturbate in a hurry, by ourselves, or with other, equally inexperienced boys. None of these circumstances are conducive to developing real sensitivity—or much skill—so we offer a few pointers.

EXPERIENCE YOUR OWN PLEASURE. If you choose to use pornography or erotica to get aroused, try, once you are aroused, to shift your focus to the sensations in your body. Pornography, though it can increase your sexual energy, is also distracting and can make it difficult for you to focus on your own sensations as you approach orgasm. Many men learn to self-pleasure with pornography, and although this is not the place to discuss the pros and cons of the First Amendment or the sex industry, it is important to recognize that pornography succeeds when it takes you away from yourself. In this practice you need to go inward and experience your own pleasure, not someone else's idea of pleasure.

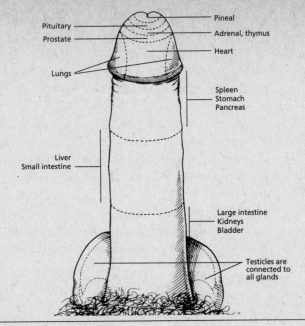

Pituitary
Prostate
Lungs
Pineal
Adrenal, thymus
Heart
Spleen
Stomach
Pancreas
Liver
Small intestine
Large intestine
Kidneys
Bladder
Testicles are
connected to
all glands

FIGURE 7. PENIS REFLEXOLOGY

STIMULATE YOUR ENTIRE PENIS. *It is important to try to stimulate your entire penis.* Most men focus primarily on the head of their penis, which is the most erogenous part. However, according to Chinese medicine, the different parts of the penis correspond to different parts of the body (see figure 7). To avoid overstimulating one part of your body, try to rub your entire penis, the shaft as well as the head.

TOUCH YOUR BALLS. If touching your scrotum is not part of your regular routine, you may want to try it. The testicles can be especially sensitive to light touch, although many men also enjoy pulling on their scrotum. Rubbing your testicles actually increases the production of testosterone, which adds to your potency both by raising your sperm count and by improving your overall health (see the Testicle Massage exercise in chapter 8). In the next section we describe the Scrotal Tug, which can help delay ejaculation, but for now you should learn to touch your scrotum just for pleasure.

EXPLORE THE MILLION-DOLLAR POINT. As you masturbate, you should explore your perineum and the Million-Dollar Point (just in front of your anus). Pushing on this spot when you are about to ejaculate can help stop the ejaculatory reflex, but again, for now you are just exploring it for its pleasure. Pushing on this spot can squeeze more blood into your penis, which will make it throb pleasurably. Strong rhythmic pressure here also imitates the prostate contractions that accompany contractile-phase orgasm.

The Million-Dollar Point is best stimulated after you have an erection and are highly aroused, since once again the body gets aroused and swells from front to back. If you do not feel any sensation or it feels uncomfortable, stop until you are more fully aroused. If you don't warm to this spot as a place of sexual stimulation, you can return to focusing on your penis and scrotum.

TAKE TIME. It is important to take as much time as you have to enjoy and learn to prolong ejaculation. "In our work with over a thousand cases," Hartman and Fithian report, "we've found that if a man can learn to go for fifteen to twenty minutes during masturbation or pleasuring, he can go as long as he wants to during intercourse. That period (fifteen to twenty minutes) seems to be critical. Once you've passed it, you have control. It's that simple."

This may seem like a long time, and it is, especially if you have been used to two- or three-minute masturbatory quickies. One multi-orgasmic man explained the difference: "When I used to play with myself, I would jack off in three to five minutes just to release tension or because I was bored or whatever. Self-cultivation is different. I try to play with myself as long as I can and not come. After a while, I could play with myself for twenty minutes." Once you become multi-orgasmic, you will be able to peak many times (without ejaculating) during these twenty or so minutes and you will be able to circulate rejuvenating, healing energy through your body. As another multi-orgasmic man described self-cultivation, "It's somewhere between masturbation and meditation."

The last thing we want to do is make pleasuring yourself mechanical or turn it into a burden, and as with lovemaking there is no one right amount of time or number of orgasms. Both depend on the situation, your free time, and your level of arousal. If you start to feel bored, ask yourself what is causing the boredom. Are you falling back into old patterns? Is your touch becoming mechanical? Are you focusing too much on your genitals? Are you distracted? If you are unable to concentrate, try the breathing exercise described in the next chapter to reconnect with your body.

Sensitizing our bodies and pampering ourselves is not something we generally consider very manly, but pleasure is just as manly as pain—and a lot more fun. It will help your practice to begin by taking a hot bath (maybe with a little soothing sesame or olive oil) and even massaging your body. Lowering the lights and lighting a candle can help you focus. You can also sit in front of a mirror (with or without a candle) and notice what your body looks like. Try to find its sensuality. Touch and feel your hands and arms, your feet (if you can reach them), calves, and thighs. Touch your chest and even your nipples. When you pleasure yourself, try massaging your thighs and stomach before you zero in on your genitals.

CULTIVATE LOVE. While most men do self-pleasure (feeling guilty or not), few are really able to do it lovingly, to cultivate love—make love to themselves—while they are doing it. Cultivating self-love is essential to being a loving partner. Sexual energy simply magnifies the energy in your body, positive or negative. If you are feeling love, love will be increased by your sexual desire. If it's hate you're feeling, then hate will be increased. It is essential that you understand the way sexual energy amplifies your emotions for both your solo and your duo practice. Cultivating your sexual energy into loving-kindness will also help you not to ejaculate; it is much more difficult to maintain control when you are feeling anger or impatience.

In Taoist sexuality you cannot separate your genitals from your heart because the sexual energy circulates throughout your entire body. As one multi-orgasmic man explained, "I used to actually want to keep sex and emotions separate, but as I practiced Taoist sexuality, my genitals became more connected to my heart and I discovered real, profound love for my partner and even for other people."

The Taoists have a simple exercise for connecting your heart and your genitals (love and sex). Try it if you find that you are feeling irritable, frustrated, or distracted when you start being sexual with yourself or your partner: put your right hand on your groin and your left hand on your heart, connecting sexual energy with love. If you often feel anger, hatred, or other negative emotions, you must transform these feelings before cultivating your sexual energy. The Inner Smile and the Six Healing Sounds—techniques described in Mantak Chia's *Taoist Ways to Transform Stress into Vitality*—can help, as can psychological counseling.

Self-love, which is quite different from egotism or narcissism, is the basis for any solo or duo practice. In *The G Spot,* the authors caution that they have not written a book about love. Our book is also not about love; it is primarily about sex. But the Taoists knew that if you are to stay healthy you can never really separate the two.

Now try a self-pleasuring exercise that will help you expand your sensual focus and extend pleasure to your entire body. In the next section, you will learn more demanding exercises for controlling your arousal and becoming multi-orgasmic. But they are based on your being highly aware of your pleasure, so we begin here with self-pleasuring.

If you are able to experience the involuntary PC contractions that occur at contractile-phase orgasm without ejaculating, you have already taken the right road to becoming a multi-orgasmic man. If you actually have two of these mini-orgasms, you already are! These will not be earth-shattering orgasms at first, but eventually they will spread throughout your body. For now just enjoy the shivering feeling of these mini-orgasms. One multi-orgasmic man described his experience: "Just as I am about to reach the point of ejaculation, I stop and relax and breathe. It's almost as if I am letting myself go or fall back into a nonejaculatory orgasm. Sometimes it feels like a pleasurable twitch in my prostate. Other times I can feel it throughout my whole genitals and it's as intense—more intense—than an ejaculatory orgasm. My wife often can't tell whether I have ejaculated or not until I tell her."

If you have not yet started to feel the contractile-phase orgasm, and if the pressure in your pelvis feels uncomfortable, you can try

EXERCISE 5

SELF-PLEASURING

1. Start by lubricating your penis. Lubricant will increase your sensations. Oil is generally better than lotion, which dries up more quickly.

2. Pleasure yourself however you like, remembering to massage and stimulate your entire penis, your scrotum, and your perineum, including the Million-Dollar Point.

3. Try to notice your increasing levels of arousal: notice the tingling at the root of your penis, notice the stages of erection, notice your heartbeat rise.

4. When you are getting near ejaculation, stop and rest. Try to notice the contraction of your PC muscle and anus that occurs at contractile-phase orgasm, although don't be surprised if it takes some time to experience this without ejaculating. You can also try to squeeze your PC muscle around your prostate if the prostate starts contracting and you are afraid you might fall over the edge.

5. After you regain control, you can start again as many times as you like and continue for as long as you like.

the Pelvic Massage exercise described later in this chapter or you can just ejaculate. Drawing the sexual energy away from your pelvis and massaging your pelvis will help decrease the pressure that all men feel when they begin. Also, if you crest over accidentally, don't give yourself a hard time. You are just beginning to learn the practice and to gain control of your arousal rate.

Learning to Control Ejaculation

Now that you have started learning how to control your breath and your sex muscles, you are ready to learn some specific techniques for controlling ejaculation when you are highly aroused. The more you practice the exercises you've learned so far, the easier it will be to practice the ones given later in this chapter and stop yourself from going past the "point of no return."

STOPPING

First, and most important, you need to stay aware of your arousal rate and *stop a few strokes* (or thrusts, if you're with your partner) before you think you will ejaculate. Many sexologists call this *the stop/start technique*, but it is just common sense. Better to stop too soon than too late. In the beginning, you will probably need to stop stimulating yourself for ten or twenty seconds to allow the urge to ejaculate to subside.

BREATHING

The deep breathing we described earlier is extremely important in controlling your arousal rate and in delaying ejaculation when you are highly aroused. One technique that has proved especially effective is to breathe in deeply and hold your breath for several moments until the urge to ejaculate subsides. Some multi-orgasmic men, however, breathe rapidly to delay ejaculation. (This quick, shallow breathing is called *the breath of fire* in the yoga tradition.) Deep, slow breathing helps control your sexual energy, whereas shallow, rapid breathing helps disperse the energy. You can experiment and see what works for you.

CONTRACTING THE PC MUSCLE

As already mentioned, the PC muscle surrounds the prostate, through which your semen must pass during the expulsion phase of orgasm. By learning to squeeze your prostate during contractile-phase orgasm (when it is contracting involuntarily), you can help yourself avoid moving from contraction to expulsion. (Between contraction and expulsion lies the infamous "point of no return.") One multi-orgasmic man described his experience: "I hold back the ejaculation simply by contracting the PC muscle at precisely the right time. It took quite some time to master this process, but the results are definitely worth the effort."

SQUEEZING THE PENIS

Many sexologists recommend squeezing the penis, a technique that was originally developed for men who ejaculate "prematurely."

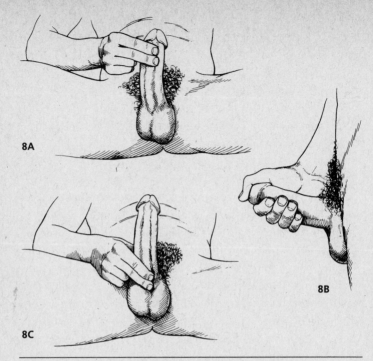

FIGURE 8. DELAYING EJACULATION WITH THE SQUEEZING METHOD

It is simple. Just place the first two fingers of either hand on the underside of your penis, place your thumb on the top, and squeeze (see figure 8a). Some men also find that gripping their penis like the handlebar of a bicycle and pressing down on the tip or underside with their thumb helps them reduce their arousal (see figure 8b). Although these techniques can be effective in solo practice, they are awkward when having intercourse because you must withdraw. To prepare for this situation, you can try using your mind to help squeeze the tip of your penis. Eventually, you will be able to squeeze the tip of your penis with just your mind and will avoid the clumsiness of having to use your hands. Another good technique is squeezing at the base of your penis (remembering to also squeeze with your mind). This will help you control your arousal and will also expand and strengthen your erections (see figure 8c).

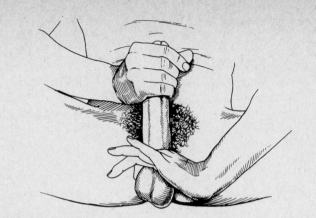

FIGURE 9. SCROTAL TUG

PRESSING THE MILLION-DOLLAR POINT

One of the oldest Taoist techniques is pressing the Million-Dollar Point while contracting your PC muscle. This helps delay ejaculation both by focusing your attention and by interrupting the ejaculatory reflex. It is simple and effective. First locate your Million-Dollar Point, which is just in front of your anus (see figure 2 on p. 12). There should be an indentation when you push at the correct spot. You will need to push your finger in up to your first joint. One multi-orgasmic man described his experience: "Pressing on the Million-Dollar Point for a while decreases my erection slightly and the danger of ejaculating greatly." You will also be able to use this technique during intercourse without withdrawing.

SCROTAL TUGGING

Since your testicles have to pull up close to the body in order to propel the semen out of the testes, pulling them away from your body can delay ejaculation. Circle the top of your sac with your thumb and forefinger (see figure 9). Pull down firmly.

DRAWING AWAY SEXUAL ENERGY

More than any mechanical technique, the secret to stopping yourself from ejaculating is learning to pump your sexual energy

EXERCISE 6

SEPARATING ORGASM FROM EJACULATION

1. Start by lubricating your penis, as you did in the Self-Pleasuring exercise.

2. Before focusing on your genitals, remember to touch and massage the rest of your body, especially your belly, thighs, and nipples.

3. Self-pleasure however you like, remembering to stimulate your entire penis, your scrotum, and your perineum.

4. Pay close attention to your arousal rate. Once again, try to notice your increasing levels of arousal: notice the tingling at the root of your penis, notice the stages of erection, notice your breathing change and your heartbeat rise.

5. As you feel yourself getting close to the point of no return, stop, breathe, and lightly contract your PC muscle around your prostate. In addition, you also can delay your ejaculation by pressing on the Million-Dollar Point, by using the scrotal tug, by pressing on the tip of your penis, or simply by using your mind to squeeze the tip of your penis. You can experiment and see which of these techniques works best for you. Most important of all, however, is paying close attention to your arousal and stopping in time—at least a few strokes before the point of no return.

6. If you feel that your sexual energy is getting too wild and difficult to control, try to draw this energy up your spine with your mind, and squeeze and release your PC muscle several times. If you are still feeling too hot and out of control, stop for ten or twenty seconds and focus on deep breathing.

7. Try to notice the contraction of your PC muscle and anus that occurs at contractile-phase orgasm.

8. After you have peaked several times without ejaculating, stop. You will feel peaceful and/or energized afterward. Try to notice your sexual energy circulating in your body, which you will feel as a tingling, itching, or prickling.

away from your genitals and up through your spine to the rest of your body. If the sexual energy continues to build up in your groin, it will eventually be too great to control and will shoot out in the most direct way it can—through your penis. However, if you draw this energy away, it will be much easier to stop yourself from ejaculating. As we discussed in the previous chapter, this is also the secret to learning how to have whole-body orgasms. In the next section we will give step-by-step instructions to show you how to circulate your sexual energy through your body. In the meantime, simply imagine drawing your sexual energy out of your penis, past your perineum, and up your spine. Contracting your perineum will help pump the energy up and will prepare you for the Big Draw exercise we describe later in this chapter.

In exercise 6, you will use these techniques to help cool you down as you start to get highly aroused. Again, you will try to experience the pleasurable involuntary pumping of the prostate and anus (contractile-phase orgasms) without ejaculating. One multi-orgasmic man described how he is able to orgasm without ejaculating: "I do a number of things. [1] Variation seems to help, not doing the same over and over again—varying the depth of the thrust when I am making love, or using different strokes when it's just me and my hand. [2] Slowing down when I feel close to the edge. [3] Deep-breathing exercises. And [4] moving the accumulated *chi* up my spine and through the Microcosmic Orbit."

Whatever techniques you use to heat yourself up and cool yourself down, *the most important parts of the practice are breathing, squeezing your* PC *muscle, and learning to relax into a nonejaculatory orgasm.*

FINDING THE WAY

Pelvic Pressure

Pressure in your pelvic area is a natural result of the increased blood and *chi* that have been pumped to the area and your increased sexual energy. If the pressure feels uncomfortable, go on and ejaculate or use deep breathing, PC Pull-Ups, and perineum massage (which we describe later in this chapter in the section called "The Finger

Lock") to relieve the tension. As you learn to feel your prostate pulsate and to draw your sexual energy up, you will be far less likely to experience pressure in your genitals (often called *blue balls*). One multi-orgasmic man described his experience: "When I stop, my penis will often stay hard for a couple more minutes, but I am not tense or uncomfortable. I don't get blue balls, because I do deep breathing and draw the energy up. I just feel relaxed."

Learning to Control Your Sexual Energy

In the next section you are going to learn the Cool Draw, the Taoist technique for drawing your sexual energy out of your testicles and circulating it through the body *before* you get hot and bothered. In the following section, you will learn the Big Draw, which you can do once you are already hot and bothered. However, it is much easier for you to work with your sexual energy when it is still "cool," and we therefore strongly encourage you to learn this exercise before attempting the Big Draw. If you learn to do the Cool Draw successfully, you will rarely need to use the Big Draw. The earlier you are able to draw the sexual energy away from your genitals, the easier it will be for you to multiply and experience whole-body orgasms and, eventually, use your sexual energy for health and healing.

When you're being sexual with yourself or a partner, the Cool Draw will allow you to decrease the urge to ejaculate. When you are feeling sexual but are not interested in being sexual or not able to be, the Cool Draw will allow you to relieve the sexual "pressure" of arousal and transform this energy into greater creativity and vitality. Michael Winn explains: "I have taught this technique to thousands of Western men and found that it is the quickest and safest way for men to relieve feelings of sexual frustration and horniness as well as to increase the flow of creative energy to their heart and brain. This technique lets a man cultivate his sexual energy anytime and anyplace—standing in line at the bank, sitting in his office, or even when he wakes up in the middle of night from a sexual dream with an erection."

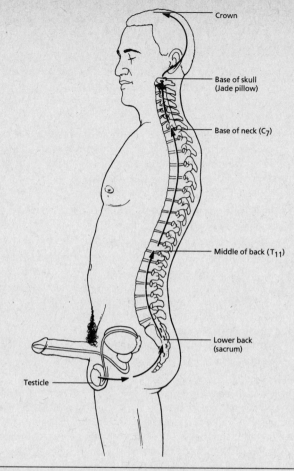

Crown

Base of skull
(Jade pillow)

Base of neck (C$_7$)

Middle of back (T$_{11}$)

Lower back
(sacrum)

Testicle

FIGURE 10. DRAWING ENERGY UP TO THE CROWN OF YOUR HEAD

The Cool Draw

The Cool Draw is also called *testicle breathing,* because the technique causes your testicles to rise and fall as if they were breathing. In actual fact, you are using your mind and muscles to raise and lower your testicles and to draw sexual energy out of your genitals and up to your brain. For Taoists, nonejaculatory orgasm allows men not only to avoid the loss of semen (and the hormones, proteins, minerals, vitamins, and amino acids it contains), but also

EXERCISE 7

THE COOL DRAW

1. *Touch or cup your testicles* with one hand to warm them up until you feel a slight tingling or the first stirring of your sexual energy. (If you are in a public place, you can simply think a sexual thought or fantasy.)

2. *Inhale and gently pull up* on the muscles around the testicles, the perineum, and the anus. As you inhale and pull your muscles up, imagine that you are sipping this sexual energy and drawing it from your testicles to your perineum and on to your anus and tailbone.

3. *Exhale and relax* your muscles, but keep your attention on your rising sexual energy.

4. *Continue to inhale and pull up and then exhale and relax* several more times until you can feel a warm or tingling sensation at your perineum. Once you are able to move this sexual energy, you can simply begin using the spine like a straw, sipping the energy from your testicles and perineum right up the entire length of your spine to the base of your skull. (Gently tucking your chin in will help the energy move from your spine into your head.) Do this for five to ten minutes or until you become aware of a light or tingling feeling in your head. With your mind, try to circle the energy in your head.

5. *Finally, touch your tongue to the roof of your mouth* half an inch behind your front teeth where the palate curves down (see figure 11). Your tongue works like a light switch that connects your front and back channels, allowing the energy to flow down the front of your body to your navel.

to avoid losing the bioelectric energy (the *ching-chi*) generated by the sperm.[6] Your testicles are the factories of your sexual hormones and sexual energy, and it is from here that you draw the energy up your spine to your brain (see figure 10). This will allow you to decrease the sexual energy in your genitals and eventually to draw a refreshing, revitalizing wave of energy up your spine, stimulating all the nerves of the body along the way. You will be able to feel this orgasmic wave of pleasure at any time without even having to be sexually aroused. That could certainly make your day—maybe even your week, your month, or your life!

DRAWING YOUR ENERGY UP

Learning to circulate this energy may take some time, so don't get discouraged, especially if you have not had much experience with meditation or other internal arts. You also may find that you feel the energy at certain points along your spine but not at others. As long as you feel the energy reach your brain, you will know that you have successfully performed the exercise.

You may be surprised to find that you are able to move this energy almost immediately. As we mentioned at the beginning of this chapter, much will depend on your sexual strength and sensitivity. One multi-orgasmic man explained his experience: "Ever since I was a teenager I have had really intense sexual energy, which has led to a lot of sexual frustration. I thought you had to be some yogi living in a cave for thirty years before you could learn to control your sexual energy. After I learned this simple exercise, I was astounded to discover that within ten minutes I was experiencing tingling in my spine and head. Within a couple of months I was able to control my continual horniness and to eliminate the feelings of frustration I had felt for so many years."

FINDING THE WAY

Loosening Up

If your back or pelvis is tight, it will be difficult for you to draw sexual energy up through your spine. It is important for you to loosen up your pelvic area, spinal column, and neck. Imagine that you are sitting on a galloping horse, and rock your pelvis back and forth, letting your chin bob up and down. Your spinal cord should rock like a wave.

DRAWING YOUR ENERGY DOWN

In addition to drawing sexual energy from the genitals up to the brain along the Back Channel, it is also essential for you to bring the energy down along the Front Channel to your belly, where it can be safely stored. This is much more difficult for men than drawing the energy up. Michael Winn explains: "A lot of men find

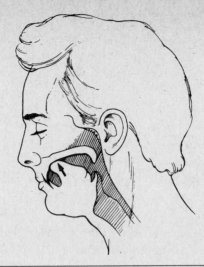

FIGURE 11. TOUCHING YOUR TONGUE TO YOUR PALATE

it is easy to bring energy up their spine. There is a connection be-tween the balls and the brain. Some even discover this pathway naturally, but most men have a harder time bringing the energy down the front where their organs are and where they uncon-sciously hold a lot of their emotional energy. Women who do the practice usually have an easier time drawing the energy down the front and may have more difficulty drawing it up the spine. In a few cases I have encountered men who find it easier to draw the sexual energy up the Front Channel, in which case I recommend that they simply circulate in the reverse direction."

Although each step helps move the energy up, *contracting your anus is the most important part of the practice because it is this squeezing action that literally pumps the energy up your spine.* Even-tually, you will be able to rely on your mind and a quick squeeze of your anus alone to bring the energy to your head.

At first you will be working on drawing the energy up to your head, which will help you experience a "brain" or whole-body or-gasm and feel energized. However, it is equally important that you draw the energy down to your navel to keep yourself balanced and to allow your body to store the energy for later use (see figure 12).

The Taoists knew the truth of the expression "What goes up must come down."

Westerners often joke about yogis who sit and contemplate their navels. Most people think the navel is simply the vestigial scar of the umbilical cord, but the navel is in fact our physical and energetic center. The navel was our first connection with the outside world: all oxygen, blood, and nutrients flowed into our fetal body through this abdominal gateway. There is an energetic reservoir at your navel where you can safely store the energy you have generated through your practice. The body can then "digest" this energy as it is needed. Also, if you are not able to raise the sexual energy all the way to the head at first, you can raise it up along your spine to your abdomen and channel it directly into this reservoir at your navel. With a little practice you should be able to draw the energy all the way up very soon.

FINDING THE WAY

What You Might Experience

I DON'T FEEL MY SEXUAL ENERGY
Unaroused sexual energy is easy to draw up and easy for your body to digest because it is not too hot. However, if you cannot feel enough sexual energy by simply touching your testicles or thinking a sexual thought, you can stimulate your genitals more directly.

I CAN'T RAISE THE ENERGY UP MY SPINE
If you are having problems drawing the energy up your spine, you can help the energy rise by using your spine's natural pumps. Your cerebrospinal fluid bathes the brain and spine. Pumps at your sacrum (the back of your pelvis) and the base of your skull help this fluid circulate and can also help you draw energy up your spine (see figure 13). These pumps, which are utilized by osteopathic physicians

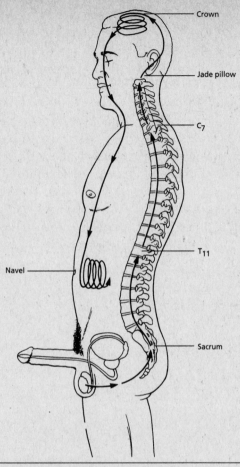

FIGURE 12. BRINGING ENERGY DOWN TO YOUR NAVEL

today, were well known to the ancient Taoists several thousand years ago. You can do the following exercise standing or sitting.

1. Activate your sacral pump by squeezing your anus up toward the tailbone and rocking your pelvis back and forth.

2. Activate your cranial pump (at the base of your skull) by drawing your chin in and up and then back out in

a soft gentle circle. Keep the jaw and neck muscles relaxed.

3. After activating the sacral and cranial pumps, rest and begin drawing the energy up your spine into your brain. Looking up with your eyes toward the top of your head will also help direct the energy up to the crown of your head. Repeatedly activate these pumps until you feel the energy move up.

I CAN'T BRING THE ENERGY DOWN

As we mentioned earlier, many men and some women have difficulty bringing the energy down. With your hands you can stroke the Front Channel along the midline of your body from your forehead down your throat and chest and to your belly. You can also try "swallowing" the energy using your saliva. (If this doesn't work, you may have a blockage in your Front Channel. See "Finding the Way: Opening Blocks in Your Front Channel" later in this chapter.)

1. Swirl your tongue around your mouth, which will activate your salivary glands.

2. Once you have a large pool of saliva, draw the sexual energy now in your brain into the saliva by focusing on the saliva. (Remember, the energy follows your mind.)

3. Swallow this pool of saliva in one gulp and follow it with your mind as it flows down your esophagus and into your stomach. Repeat this swallowing and imagine the energy collecting in a pool at your stomach.

4. Finally, with both hands stroke the front of your body from your throat straight down to your belly.

Most people today carry around a great deal of physical and emotional tension. As you are trying to circulate energy, you may notice tightness or congestion in your back or chest. Men in particular

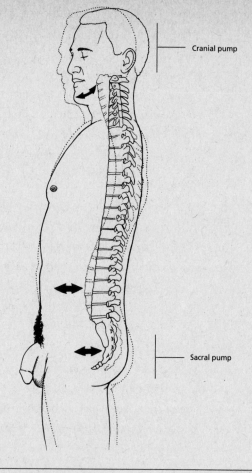

Cranial pump

Sacral pump

FIGURE 13. SACRAL AND CRANIAL PUMPS
Help the energy rise up your spine by rocking your sacrum and drawing your chin in and up.

are prone to holding in their emotions, which often can lead to energetic blockages in the Front Channel, along which emotions are stored—that is, in your heart, solar plexus, stomach, and intestines. It is essential that you open these blockages before attempting the Big Draw. (If you are still having a problem bringing the energy down, even after opening any blocks in your Front Channel, try the powerful Venting exercise described in the next section.)

Opening Blocks in Your Front Channel

If you are having difficulty drawing the energy down and suspect you might have a blockage, try the following:

1. Put your left hand on your belly and put your right hand at the base of your throat just above your heart center.

2. Imagine as you inhale that you are drawing energy up the Front Channel to your right hand and from there up your throat to the tip of your tongue.

3. As you exhale, imagine you are reversing the flow so it descends back down past your heart to your belly. This will help open any energy blocks in your Front Channel.

The Big Draw

Now that you have learned to circulate your sexual energy when it is not too aroused, you need to learn how to circulate and control this energy when it *is* aroused. Here the energy will be hotter, more explosive, and harder to keep from shooting out your penis. However, before attempting the Big Draw, you must make sure you are able to circulate your energy as described in the last exercise. Stopping aroused sexual energy is like trying to stop a team of horses who are speeding toward a cliff. Before you attempt this with the Big Draw, you must make sure you know how to ride, which is what the Cool Draw exercise teaches you.

As we mentioned in chapter 1, ejaculation is simply an involuntary muscle spasm, which you are learning to make voluntary so that you can choose if and when you want to ejaculate. Michael Winn explains how the Big Draw works: "Ejaculation can happen only if there is enough energy in the local nerves and enough blood in the local muscles to trigger the muscle spasm. There's nothing

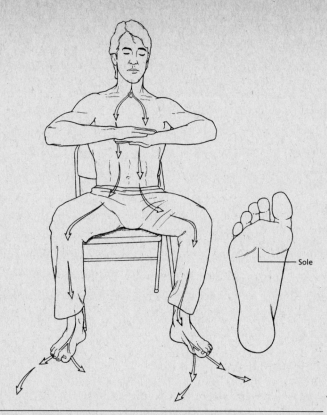

Sole

FIGURE 14. BRINGING ENERGY DOWN TO YOUR FEET AND TOES

mystical about the Big Draw technique for stopping the ejaculatory spasm. You squeeze the PC muscles around the sperm ducts and then progressively pump the big muscles in the buttocks (and, if necessary, the foot, fist, and jaw muscles). These big muscles draw the blood away from the genitals. At the same time, you draw the energy away from the genital nerves by shifting your mental focus into a wave of nerve sensations traveling up your spine into your brain. The combination of these actions simply removes the blood and energy the genital muscles need in order to involuntarily spasm. It is as simple as that. All the squeezing and clenching is a bit crude, but it works. If any man practices properly and regularly, eventually he'll get it. I have hundreds of students who have proved this."

When you begin learning the Big Draw, you will need to use the various techniques described in this section. Eventually, when doing the Big Draw you will be able to use just your mind and maybe a quick squeeze of your PC muscle. According to one multi-orgasmic man, "In the beginning, I had to contract my muscles, especially the perineum and the anus, while concentrating on drawing the energy up with my mind. Now the energy moves up almost by itself."

FINDING THE WAY

Cautions

The Big Draw is a very powerful practice, and you need to make sure you follow a few safety tips.

NEVER LEAVE SEXUAL ENERGY IN THE BRAIN FOR LONG PERIODS OF TIME

Remember to touch your tongue to your palate to allow this energy to come down through the Front Channel to the navel, where it can be safely stored. In the past, many teachers of Eastern sexuality taught students how to draw energy up to their brain without teaching them how to bring it back down again. This resulted in what has been called *the Kundalini syndrome*. The Taoists knew the importance of completing the circle. Anytime you feel like you have too much energy, inhale to your abdomen, and as you exhale, bring the energy all the way down to your toes and the soles of your feet (see figure 14).

MAKE SURE YOU ARE FEELING BALANCED

Remember that the sexual energy you will be circulating through your body will amplify any emotions you are feeling. Michael Winn explains: "The most important thing is to first try to clear out your emotional extremes and avoid practicing when you are feeling extreme anger or extreme anything." You should also avoid practicing if you are too tired. If you have a medical condition, you should speak with a Healing Tao instructor (see the appendix) before you begin this practice.

TAKE IT EASY

Although it may not seem very important, your attitude toward the practice is in fact essential. As Healing Tao instructor Walter Beckley explains, "A lot of men go into the practice gung ho, which is good, but they need to be careful not to jam the energy up their spine or they can hurt themselves. Your attitude needs to be playful and joyful. You need to be soft with your body. It is better for you to lose the energy, to ejaculate, than to try to force the energy up your spine."

PREPARE YOURSELF

Practice on an empty, but not hungry, stomach whenever possible. Always wait at least one hour after eating. The body needs energy to digest the food you have just eaten, which means there will be less energy for you to circulate. Also, wear loose clothes. Although there should be a gentle flow of clean air in the room, avoid drafts or wind. And remember to always breathe through your nose.

POSITION YOURSELF

In the beginning, do not lie on your back during these exercises, since the rising sexual energy may stick in your chest and cause pain. At first, sit, stand, or lie on your side. If you lie on your side, always do so on your right side. (Lying on the left side puts too much strain on your heart.) Once you master these exercises, you can do them in any position. Also, never place any objects (such as a pillow) under you while lying on your right side, since this will bend the channel of energy and can cause back pain.

WARNING

If you have an active herpes sore, do not do this practice until you have healed. If you have herpes but it is in remission (that is, if you have no visible sore), you can do this practice.

___

At first you will use your big muscles to help draw the energy upward. Soon you will use these muscles less and learn to rely more on your PC muscle. Eventually you will be able to concentrate your attention at the top of your head and draw the energy up effortlessly. It may take you some time to learn to do this, but eventually you will be able to direct an invigorating streak of energy up your spine just by thinking about it.

Once you have mastered the Big Draw, you will be able to draw the energy up in any situation: while you are walking, standing in line, driving your car, or lying in bed. In the beginning, however, choose a quiet time when you will not be interrupted so that you can concentrate on directing this subtle and life-giving flow of energy through your body.

Do not be concerned if you feel little effect after the first few days or even weeks of practice. Each person needs a different amount of time to learn to circulate energy in the body. If you have practiced other mental exercises such as meditation, yoga, or martial arts, you will find it easier to do these exercises. If this is your first attempt at the internal arts, don't get frustrated. It takes time to learn concentration. Though this may seem difficult, you will be amazed at how quickly you begin to notice the energy moving in your body. Since the energy flows along natural circuits, the energy guides your mind even as your mind guides the energy. And as we mentioned earlier, you will soon be able to forget about most of the steps in the exercise and just guide the energy up with your mind. But, as with driving a car, before you can forget the individual steps, you must learn them.

Pumping energy up your spine through the Big Draw works on the same principle as a water pump. By pumping your muscles, you are creating the pressure and suction to draw the energy up, but it

THE BIG DRAW

1. Stand and pleasure yourself until you have a strong erection but well before you reach the point of no return (thirty seconds to a minute before you would otherwise ejaculate).

2. Stop stimulating yourself and rest for a moment to regain control. Then simultaneously contract your PC muscle firmly *around your prostate gland* and clamp your toes down on the floor.

3. Inhale and draw your sexual energy away from the perineum toward your anus and spine by squeezing your buttocks tightly.

4. As if you were pumping the brakes on a car, contract in waves the muscles from your anus up your spine, each time taking a short inhalation. Rocking your spine back and forth as if you were riding a horse will also help the energy to move up the spine.

5. As the energy reaches the base of your skull, make sure your chin is tucked in gently to help the energy move from the spine into your head.

6. Roll your eyes up as if you were looking at the top of your head, which will help bring the energy all the way up to the crown of your head.

7. When you have pumped the energy up to the crown of your head, you have done one Big Draw. The state of your erection is a measure of how successfully you have been doing the Big Draw: as you draw the energy out of your genitals and up your spine, your erection should decrease.

8. Repeat steps 3 through 6 eight more times.

9. After you have pumped the energy up to the crown of your head nine times, use your mind, your eyes, and all your senses to spiral this creative sexual energy in your brain nine, eighteen, or thirty-six times, first in one direction, and then the other. When you have finished spiraling, rest for a while and experience the sensational feeling of energy in your brain, often felt as warmth and tingling, like a mini-orgasm.

10. When you feel that your brain is full, touch your tongue to your palate and let the energy flow down the Front Channel from your brain first to between your eyebrows, then to your nose, throat, heart, and solar plexus, and finally to your navel, where it can be stored.

is while you are relaxing that the energy will be easiest to guide up your spine. During the resting periods, your mind should stay focused on the flow of energy.

It is best to practice in the morning or afternoon, since at night the increased energy you will have after doing the Big Draw may make it difficult for you to sleep. If this happens or if you find you have too much "nervous" energy, simply touch your tongue to your palate (which will connect the Back and Front Channels) and draw the energy down from your head to your navel, where it can be stored. You can also spiral the energy in your head, as we mentioned earlier, and use the techniques you learned in the Cool Draw. If the problem of increased energy still persists, you can use the Venting exercise described later in this section.

FINDING THE WAY

What You Might Experience

I DON'T FEEL ANYTHING

We have suggested that you do the Big Draw when your sexual energy is not too aroused. The hotter it is, the more difficult it is to control and the more likely you are to ejaculate, losing the energy you are trying to draw up. However, if you do not feel enough sexual energy, arouse yourself 95 to 99 percent of the way to orgasm. Once you are able to orgasm without ejaculating, you can arouse yourself all the way to orgasm and still draw the energy up to your brain. When you are about to orgasm or are orgasming, stop, and practice the Big Draw three to nine times, or until the orgasmic feeling moves upward.

IT'S TOO HOT

You may find that your energy is too hot, too explosive, and you are either ejaculating or having a hard time drawing the energy up your spine. If that is the case, arouse yourself less.

VENTING

1. Lie down on your back. Elevate your knees with a pillow if you feel any pain in the small of your back or lumbar area.

2. Place your hands in front of your mouth so that the tips of your fingers touch and so that your palms are facing toward your feet.

3. Close your eyes and take a deep breath. Feel your stomach and chest expand gently.

4. Smile and exhale quietly, making the sound *heeeeee*. As you are exhaling, push your hands toward your feet and imagine that your body is a hollow tube that you are emptying with your hands.

5. Repeat this sound and movement three, six, or nine times, each time imagining that you are pushing this excess energy from your head, past your heart and belly, through your legs, and out your feet. You can also try the exercise while standing or sitting. If you are still having a problem venting your energy, contact a Healing Tao instructor (see the appendix) or an acupuncturist.

You need to have enough energy that you can draw it up, but at first, at least, you don't want to have too much energy.

I KEEP EJACULATING

If you get too close to the point of no return, you should try continuously contracting your PC muscle so as to firmly grasp your prostate and stop yourself from ejaculating. You can keep your PC muscle clenched while you are pumping your buttock muscles. If you are close to ejaculation and need additional force to redirect the energy up, at the same time that you squeeze your buttocks, also tighten your hands into fists and clench your jaw muscles and teeth. This will increase the pressure of your pumping action. However, this last technique should be avoided by men who store tension in their neck and jaw.

MY BACK HURTS

It is sometimes a little difficult to draw the energy into the base of the spine, and some people experience a little pain, tingling, or "pins and needles" when this energy first enters the sacrum. If this happens to you, do not be alarmed. You can help pass the energy through by gently massaging the area with your fingers.

MY EYES HURT

When you roll your eyes up or around, you may find that your eye muscles ache or your head aches. This is a typical sign of sore muscles and is nothing to worry about. If this problem persists, go easy on this part of the practice or contact a Healing Tao instructor (see the appendix).

MY HEAD HURTS

If your head hurts, you feel "wired," or you are having diffi-culty sleeping, you may be leaving too much stagnant en-ergy in your head. The energy can overheat if it stays in one place—a problem that can be easily solved by keeping the energy moving. Make sure to circulate the energy in your head nine, eighteen, or thirty-six times in one direction and then the other. (Like in cooking, you need to stir the pot so no part of the stew overcooks.) Once you have circled the energy in your head, let it flow down the front of your body through the Front Channel. If you are having a problem bringing the energy down the Front Channel, you can let it descend back down your spine.

I AM FEELING IRRITABLE AND ANGRY

In addition to amplifying anger that you may already have, the new energy can also cause you to overheat and develop negative emotions, such as anger, if you are not circulating the energy enough. In this case try to focus on recycling this anger and other negative emotions into loving-kindness. Also see the section called "When to Ejaculate" later in this chapter.

OTHER SIDE EFFECTS

A small percentage of men who try these techniques experience excess energy stuck in their upper body. Symptoms of this vary from person to person but may include insomnia, a ringing in the ears, heart palpitations, or tension headaches that persist for several days. If you have any of these symptoms, immediately stop the practice and do the Venting exercise described later in this section. If they persist, contact a Healing Tao instructor (see the appendix) or acupuncturist. Most Western doctors will not be able to correctly diagnose or treat the problem, since they are not trained to understand the movement of energy in the body and its physical effects. It is worth mentioning that the problems are not caused by the circulation of your sexual energy but by preexisting emotional and physical tensions trapped in the upper body. The sexual energy simply amplifies these problems, which is why it is essential for you to address these underlying issues before advancing further with your sexual practice.

As already mentioned, if you are having a problem drawing the energy down, you may have a block in your Front Channel. The Taoists use sounds to open up blocked energy channels and to heal the body. This technique is called the Six Healing Sounds. (A detailed description of this practice can be found in Mantak Chia's *Taoist Ways to Transform Stress into Vitality*.) The sound that will open up your Front Channel and help you vent excess energy is known as the *triple warmer* or *triple heater* sound.

After each practice session of the Big Draw, be sure to massage your genitals. This will disperse any energy that did not get drawn

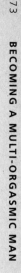

FIGURE 15.   THE FINGER LOCK

up and will alleviate any feelings of congestion or fullness. Also massage your perineum, your coccyx, and your sacrum as described in the Pelvic Massage exercise given later in this chapter. If your testicles feel full, you can also do the Testicle Massage exercise given in chapter 8. The Testicle Massage, like the Pelvic Massage, will help your body absorb sexual energy and sperm.

The Finger Lock

Now we are going to show you how to stop the semen once you are passing what Masters and Johnson call *ejaculatory inevitability*—in other words, when you are going past the point of no return. It is best to use the Big Draw whenever possible, and increasingly to use your mind to stop yourself from ejaculating rather than your fingers, which can be awkward. Use this technique when you need to conserve your energy, such as when you are sick or working hard, but have been unable to stop yourself from ejaculating. When you use the Finger Lock to block the semen from coming out once you have passed the point of no return, you will lose your erection.

EXERCISE 10

THE FINGER LOCK

1. When you feel that ejaculation is inevitable, press the three middle fingers (in other words, not your pinkie or thumb) of your dominant hand into the Million-Dollar Point just hard enough to stop the flow of semen.

2. Your fingers should be curved slightly and your middle finger should push directly against the urethral tube. This tube expands when you near ejaculation, so it should be easy to find. Your other two fingers should press on each side of the tube to hold it in place.

3. Contract your PC muscle, which encircles the prostate, and pull up your perineum. Draw the orgasmic energy up to the spine and to your brain.

4. Hold your fingers in place before, during, and after the contractions.

5. When the pumping has stopped completely, remove your fingers.

However, you may find that it returns more quickly. One multi-orgasmic man explained: "After using the Finger Lock I could get an erection and have sex again very soon."

In the last section we discussed the Million-Dollar Point as a place where you could press to delay ejaculation. The Million-Dollar Point is also the place where you can actually block the semen from leaving your body once you have passed the point of no return. One multi-orgasmic man described when it was that he found the Finger Lock most helpful: "In the beginning I used the Finger Lock during self-cultivation. I could train myself to go closer and closer to the point of no return because I could use it if I went over. I would recommend practicing it first in self-cultivation so it is not awkward during lovemaking."

Basically, the Finger Lock involves pressing the Million-Dollar Point, the indentation directly in front of your anus, with the three middle fingers of your right hand (see figure 15). If you're a lefty, use your left hand; you will need the strength of your dominant hand to use this technique. (Also, make sure your fingernails are cut short and filed so you don't hurt yourself.) You need to press here just as you feel yourself passing the point of no return—but before you actually start ejaculating—and to continue pressing until the ejaculatory contractions stop.

You will be pushing down on the spot where the ejaculatory duct and the membranous urethra meet. One multi-orgasmic man suggests: "You should realize that the concentration and pressure that you need during your orgasm will reduce your enjoyment of the orgasmic contractions in the beginning. Knowing this, you will better be able to continue applying the pressure to the end." Not to worry: this will get easier and less distracting with time.

If you're applying pressure to the right place, no semen will come out. If semen does come out, you have not yet found your Million-Dollar Point. Try moving your fingers slightly closer to the anus next time, and make sure you are pushing firmly into the indentation.

If you are curious to see whether you did the exercise correctly, you can urinate into a cup. If the urine is clear, you are doing it right. If the urine is very cloudy, the semen went into your bladder in a retrograde ejaculation. If this happened, the next time (as we mentioned already) try moving your three fingers back slightly toward your anus.

When you block the semen with your fingers, most of the fluid returns to the epididymis and the seminal vesicles. The tissues in this region are extremely elastic and are not harmed by this technique, but it is very important after this exercise to massage the pelvic areas (see the Pelvic Massage exercise on page 76), to do PC Pull-Ups, and, ideally, to circulate your sexual energy through your body, as described in the previous section. You may feel some pressure or even pain when you begin using the Finger Lock, which will mean it is all the more important to help your body reabsorb the semen. One multi-orgasmic man explained his experience: "You have to be careful with the Finger Lock not to push too hard. One night my pumpers were starting to pump and I really pressed hard, but it hurt afterward for a while."

You can relieve much of the pressure you may feel in your pelvis after using the Finger Lock or Big Draw by massaging several key points in your pelvic area. First and most important is to massage your perineum (the spot between the root of your penis and your anus) and testicles (for the Testicle Massage exercise, see chapter

PELVIC MASSAGE

1. Using your fingers, massage your Million-Dollar Point in a circle, first in one direction and then the other.

2. Repeat this massage between your anus and tailbone.

3. Repeat this massage at each of the eight holes of the sacrum. If you can't find the individual holes, massage the general area in several different places, circling first in one direction and then the other.

8). This will relieve a lot of the pressure and help your body re-absorb the semen. It is also important to massage your tailbone—specifically, where there is an indentation between your anus and your tailbone (see figure 16) and the eight holes of your sacrum (see figure 17). This will help your body absorb the sexual energy you have generated.

FINDING THE WAY

Pain

If you have intense pain, you are probably pushing too far forward or too late. When this happens, the urethra, which is like a hose that has been pinched, swells up with fluid and can hurt. You need to turn off the faucet before the water (or, in this case, semen) enters the hose. Make sure you push farther back and/or sooner next time. Also make sure you are not pushing too hard. Some discomfort is common, especially during the first few weeks, from the pressure you apply with your fingers and the fluid pressure in your pelvis, but it shouldn't hurt for long. If you are experiencing pain, try to refine the technique or forget this stop-gap measure and learn the more important Big Draw.

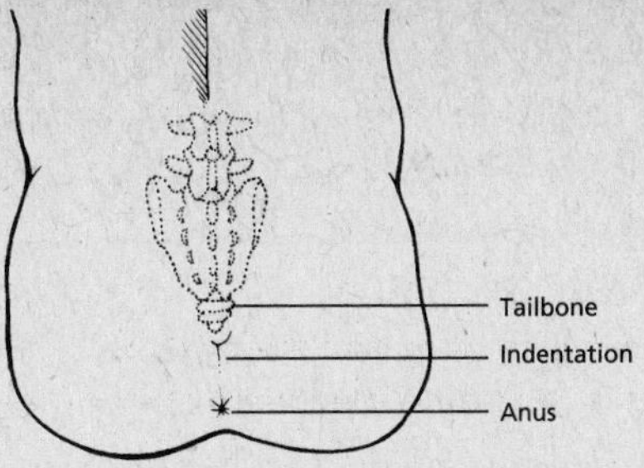

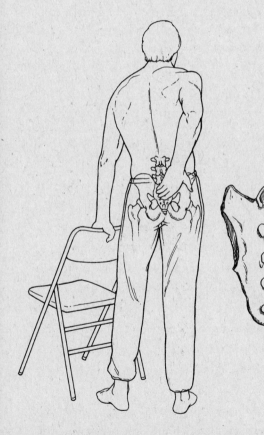

Tailbone
Indentation
Anus

FIGURE 16. MASSAGING THE INDENTATION BETWEEN THE TAILBONE AND ANUS

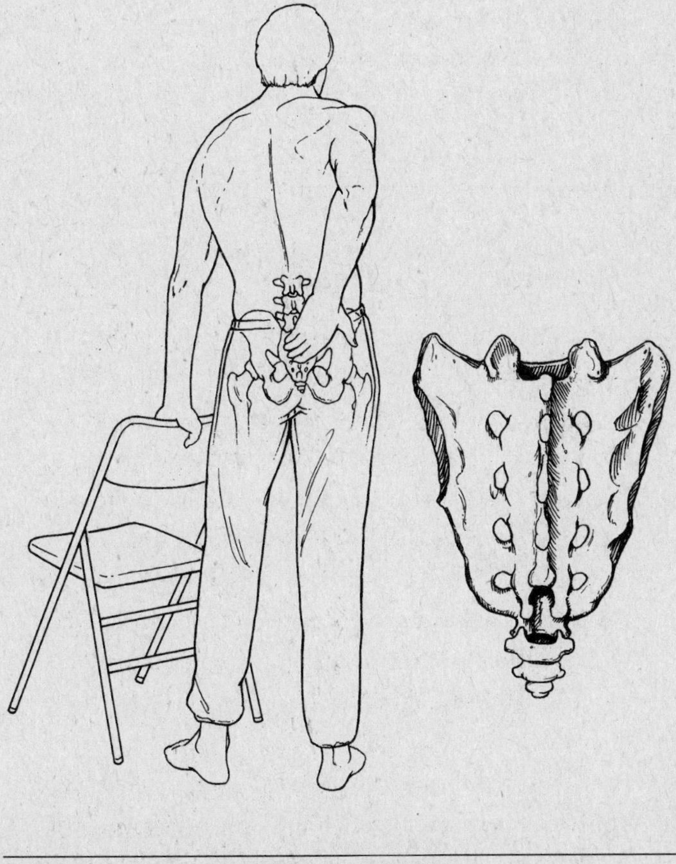

FIGURE 17. MASSAGING THE HOLES OF THE SACRUM

A small amount of semen will leak out once you lose your erection, so this is not a method of birth control or safe sex. Using it with other forms of contraception, however, will improve their effectiveness. Since you still lose some of your energy with this technique, the sooner you are able to learn the Big Draw, the better off you will be. Although at first you may feel fatigued, your energy will return sooner than if you had ejaculated.

This is a powerful practice, which you should not use more than once every two or three days when you start. If you are elderly or ill, you should not use this practice more than twice a week when you begin. The retained sexual energy may cause you to feel hot or thirsty. If so, try drinking more water. After you have practiced this technique for one to three months, and sometimes sooner, you will notice your sex drive increase and your erections become more frequent. Increase your sexual activities (solo and duo) moderately; try not to overdo it.

FINDING THE WAY

Pressure in Your Head

After a month or more of practice, you may find that you feel pressure in your head, a result of the increased energy in your body. This is a sign of progress, that your body has more energy than before. For some this can be experienced as a pleasurable tingling, like static electricity without the shock. (This is the same Kundalini energy popularized by Tantric teachers in the West.) However, if this power grows uncomfortable, it once again can be circulated to the rest of the body by pressing your tongue to the roof of your mouth and letting the energy flow down.

If you have high blood pressure, you should keep your tongue in your lower jaw (rather than touching your palate) and also bring the energy all the way down to the soles of your feet (see figure 14). Physical exercise, massaging your feet, and a heavy grain diet will also help you ground the energy. If you are not ready to learn how to circulate your sexual energy, you can simply ejaculate once or twice to release the extra energy.

When to Stop

Most men stop masturbating or having sex when they ejaculate, but after you learn the Big Draw and become multi-orgasmic, you may be faced with the very real question of when to stop. There will be days when you want to self-pleasure or make love for a long time, and there will be other days when you want a satisfying multi-orgasmic quickie. The choice is really yours and will depend on what is happening in your life. Your and your partner's desire and satisfaction should guide you.

It is important, however, not to overdo it, especially at first. As senior Healing Tao instructor Masahiro Ouchi explains, "Men feel very powerful when they start practicing Sexual Kung Fu, and often they don't know when to stop. Take it slow, and let your body and your partner adjust." You will also need to make sure your partner has enough sexual strength to keep up with the new intensity in your lovemaking. You can encourage her to read chapter 6, which is written especially for her, but try not to push her, and be sensitive to her needs. You can always practice on your own.

Many people worry about masturbating too much or think that they will neglect other parts of their life if they let themselves experience too much pleasure. According to the Tao, if you are able to pleasure and satisfy yourself, you will not need to constantly run after superficial sex or other unsatisfying stimulation.

FINDING THE WAY

Let Your Erection Decrease Every Twenty Minutes

If you regularly pleasure yourself or make love for more than twenty minutes—which you very well may do after you become multi-orgasmic—*it is important to let your erection decrease somewhat about every twenty minutes to allow the blood to recirculate through the body.* It is worth mentioning again that Sexual Kung Fu is not an endurance test. Pleasure and cultivate yourself as long as you have the time and the desire.

When to Ejaculate

Every time you orgasm, you draw more sexual energy into your body; therefore, if you eventually ejaculate, you lose less energy than you would have had you not had multiple orgasms beforehand. For example:

1. If you have half a dozen orgasms (each time circulating the energy to your brain and the rest of your body) and then ejaculate, you will lose about 50 percent of your sexual energy.
2. If you have half a dozen orgasms and then use the Finger Lock, you will lose about a quarter of your sexual energy.
3. If you have half a dozen orgasms and then use the Big Draw (and don't ejaculate), you will not lose any of your sexual energy.

The final option will give you the greatest opportunity to cultivate the ecstatic orgasms that you feel in your brain and throughout your body. It will also allow you to cultivate this energy for your overall health. However, by generating and containing this much energy, you risk overheating unless you are able to circulate the energy through the Microcosmic Orbit.

FINDING THE WAY

Preventing Overheating

According to the Tao, erection energy is wood (or liver) energy. So when you don't ejaculate and you pull up the orgasmic energy, you will increase this energy in your liver. If this increasing energy is not transformed into love and kindness, it will transform into anger and hatred. So when you have a lot of energy, practice being especially kind and loving to your partner or, if you do not have a partner, to other people in your life.

Other techniques for preventing yourself from overheating include drinking a lot of water and even swallowing your own saliva, which has a cooling effect on the body. Your emotional state can also affect the energy in your body. If you feel calm and loving, the body can much more easily absorb the energy. If you feel anger or disdain for yourself or your partner, you run a greater risk of overheating. If you are overheating or feel you have more energy than you can absorb, you should probably ejaculate. If the problem persists, try practicing the Inner Smile or the Six Healing Sounds described in *Taoist Ways to Transform Stress into Vitality,* or contact a Healing Tao instructor (see the appendix).

The Taoist ideal is to ejaculate as infrequently as you can, but every man can and should refrain from ejaculating for a period of time suited to him. In the words of Su Nü, "One must measure one's own strength and ejaculate accordingly. Anything else is simply force and foolishness." Your strength depends on your age, your health, your state of mind, and your willpower.

Sun Ssu-miao, one of the leading physicians of ancient China, recommended that *men attain good health and longevity by ejaculating twice a month,* as long as they ate healthily and exercised. He also offered the following more specific guidelines.

A man at *twenty* can ejaculate once every *four* days.
A man at *thirty* can ejaculate once every *eight* days.
A man at *forty* can ejaculate once every *ten* days.
A man at *fifty* can ejaculate once every *twenty* days.
A man at *sixty* should *no longer ejaculate.*

It goes without saying that his prescription did not limit the number of times a man of any age could have sex and nonejaculatory orgasms. This restriction on ejaculation may sound like a disappointment, but once you have had multiple nonejaculatory orgasms, you won't miss ejaculating at all. In the words of one multi-orgasmic man, "Once you have multi's [non-ejaculatory orgasms], you never want to go back to squirt [ejaculatory] orgasms. Squirt orgasms are just in your genitals; multi's are whole-body orgasms."

Sun Ssu-miao, who lived to 101, ejaculated only after making love one hundred times. But rather than adhering to any rigid numerical formula, you should try to pay attention to your body. If you are exhausted or sick, drunk or stuffed with food, you should avoid ejaculating. If you are working hard you will want to conserve your semen, but if you are on vacation you may wish to ejaculate a little more often. The ancient Taoists, who lived close to nature, also believed that just as plants and animals conserve their energy in winter, so should people. Besides the seasons, there are other rhythms that will determine the number of times you ejaculate. If you are trying to conceive a child, you will need to ejaculate whenever your partner is ovulating.

In general, when you ejaculate you should feel refreshed and energetic. If ejaculating leaves you feeling empty, depressed, or exhausted, you need to increase the amount of time between ejaculations or avoid ejaculating altogether until you build up your sexual energy. When you do ejaculate, you can conserve some semen and sexual energy by approaching the point of no return slowly rather than thrusting vigorously to a climax. After you ejaculate, you can also practice PC contractions to tighten your pelvic muscles and reduce the amount of energy that typically leaks out after ejaculation.

At the same time it is important not to become obsessive about nonejaculation and not to give yourself a hard time when you do ejaculate. As Michael Winn explains, "It is very important not to be fanatical about nonejaculation. A lot of men who learn about Sexual Kung Fu think, 'Wow, this is great. It makes sense. I want to do it.' And then they have a problem controlling their ejaculation. And then they start passing judgment on themselves and feeling guilty. They are missing the point, which is not even whether you ejaculate or not, but whether you are able to recycle some of the sexual energy up through your body before you ejaculate. Obviously, the longer you can delay your ejaculation, the greater your opportunity to cultivate this energy for creative and spiritual growth. *If you need to ejaculate and it's coming and you can't stop it, just go for it. Don't beat yourself up. Because what is really important ultimately is not just the energy in the sperm, but the overall love between you and your partner.*"

Remember that the energy is more than just the sperm: if you are able to draw any energy out of the sperm, you are far ahead of where you were before you started, in terms both of the level of pleasure you will be able to experience and of the energy you will be able to circulate for your health. True sexual satisfaction comes from both pleasure and health; in the next chapter, we show you how to share both of these with your partner.

POWER AND SEXUALITY

The practices that you are learning in this book are very powerful, and once you learn them it is natural for you to be proud of your ability to master your sexual energy and of your newfound skill in bed. However, it is essential that you avoid the bravado and machismo that accompany so much male sexuality. As Senior Healing Tao instructor Masahiro Ouchi explains, "Sexual Kung Fu is quite easy to learn, and many men start feeling very powerful in bed, but it must not become a power trip. Power is about conquest, which is the opposite of love and any real spiritual practice." Ouchi, who holds a black belt in karate, compares Sexual Kung Fu to what he has observed in karate: "Most people who have black belts use this power incorrectly. They become more rigid and egotistical and lose the sensitivity and gentleness that are the real source of this power."

To practice Sexual Kung Fu correctly, you need to open your heart and practice with a spirit of humility and loving-kindness, not arrogance and self-centeredness. Egotism is just an expression of insecurity, and as you learn real sexual confidence, you will be able to let go of pretension and posturing. Remember that this practice and your new sexual energy will magnify your emotions, so it is essential that you cultivate them. If arrogance and egotism are problems for you, try to practice the Six Healing Sounds (see *Taoist Ways to Transform Stress into Vitality*). If you do not address these emotions, they will limit your practice, your pleasure, and your partnership.

THE ART OF LOVEMAKING

Many men who begin practicing Sexual Kung Fu get so involved with their own practice that they lose touch with their partner and with the spontaneous and ecstatic process of lovemaking. You can practice as often as you want on your own, but when you are with your partner, it is extremely important to remember that it is not just *your* practice. The point of lovemaking is to make love, and from this love come pleasure and health; it is not about generating sexual energy for yourself or demonstrating your skill. As Masahiro Ouchi explains, "The technique is just that—technique. It is not the real art. You need to learn the technique well enough that you can forget about it. Just like playing a musical instrument, at first you need to learn the scales, but then you need to forget about them and just play from the heart." In the next two chapters we move from the solo-cultivation exercises that help you become a multi-orgasmic man to the duo-cultivation exercises that help you and your partner become a multi-orgasmic couple. (Gay men may wish to skip directly to chapter 7.)

CHAPTER FOUR

Know Your Partner

"Among the skills possessed by men, a knowledge of women is indispensable," explains *Discourse on the Highest Tao Under Heaven*. "When one does have a woman, only the skillful are equal to the task." The union of man and woman has been the foundation of Sexual Kung Fu, for through this primal bond, it was believed, infinite pleasure and priceless health could be attained. With this incentive, the Taoists refined lovemaking into a high art of intimacy and ecstasy.

A harmonious love life was considered essential to conjugal happiness, and newlyweds were given "pillow books" that graphically demonstrated how they could achieve this bliss. We would never think of learning to cook without some guidance or a cookbook or two, but in lovemaking, which is certainly as complex as cooking, Western men and women are forced to discover for themselves the mysterious world of sex with only a few hopelessly romanticized images from the movies and television to guide them.

Hollywood sex is not good sex; it is just fast sex. The passionate, urgent embrace portrayed in most films in which the woman is instantly lubricated and immediately satisfied by a few minutes of coital writhing would be laughable if it did not leave so many viewers trying to imitate this unrealistic model of lovemaking. It is worth remembering that the director's imperative of keeping the plot moving, and the public's intolerance for watching the body in pleasure, make it impossible to explore on-screen the subtle nuances of lovemaking. Candace Bergen described her formula for cinematic orgasms in *Esquire* magazine: "Ten seconds of heavy breathing, roll your head from side to side, simulate a slight asthma attack, and die a little." So much for foreplay.

Porn films, in which the "plot" is generally just celluloid glue between the sex scenes, should offer the opportunity to learn a richer sexual repertoire. However, the frantic, nonstop thrusting in most pornography is timed more to the masturbatory stroke of a man's hand than to the subtle and profound sensations of real flesh-and-blood lovemaking.

It is no wonder that Western men, weaned on movies, television, and porn, ejaculate so quickly. Almost 80 percent of the men Kinsey studied ejaculated less than two minutes after entering their partner. Both men and women may lose out in this rapid-fire coitus. Hartman and Fithian speculate that this quick intercourse does not allow enough time for the natural chemicals that accompany touch and sexual arousal to be released into the bloodstream, short-circuiting the general sense of well-being that usually accompanies lovemaking. The Taoists would say that in such hasty sex the man and woman are not able to exchange sexual energy and to harmonize with one another, and may even drain each other of energy. This does not mean that quickies are not sometimes just what the doctor ordered, especially if you and your partner have a practice of ecstatic lovemaking that allows you to harmonize and satisfy each other quickly.

Almost a quarter century after Kinsey published his findings—in the wake of the sexual revolution and women's liberation—Morton Hunt found in a follow-up study that men were lasting ten minutes instead of two. Though still rather short by Taoist standards, this increase is a 400 percent improvement nonetheless. Although men are generally portrayed as insensitive lovers, guided in bed exclusively by their own self-interest, clearly a major motivation for men learning to last longer in bed in recent years has been their desire to pleasure their partners, who were beginning to discover that they could be orgasmic or even multi-orgasmic. In interviews with four thousand men, Anthony Pietropinto found that a surprising 80 percent judged their own sexual satisfaction by whether they had been able to give their partner one or more orgasms.[1] Once you are multi-orgasmic, you will be able to satisfy your partner no matter how long she takes to orgasm.

In learning to satisfy your partner, however, the first thing you must do is remove your ego. You are not "giving" her an orgasm. You are not trying to be the best lover she has ever had. Too many men get caught up with sexual performance. If you are able to replace performance with pleasure—hers and yours—you will be able to satisfy even the lustiest of lovers. Remember, the best lovers are men who are completely relaxed and aware of what is going on in both their own and their partner's bodies. In chapter 2, you began learning how to understand what happens in your body, and in this chapter you will learn how to recognize what is happening in your lover's.

There is one last point worth keeping in mind. It is much easier to practice Sexual Kung Fu with a regular partner with whom you have a deep emotional as well as physical bond. In their study of multi-orgasmic men, Dunn and Trost found that it was much easier for men to become multi-orgasmic with a familiar partner with whom there was emotional closeness and the opportunity for leisurely sex. Each man they interviewed mentioned that the goal was not to have multiple orgasms but to have pleasurable and satisfying lovemaking. Multiple orgasms are just one of the many treasures you will discover along the path to intimate and ever more ecstatic lovemaking.

Her Body

Women's sexuality has been the source of much mystery and mystification throughout Western history. Women's largely internal (as

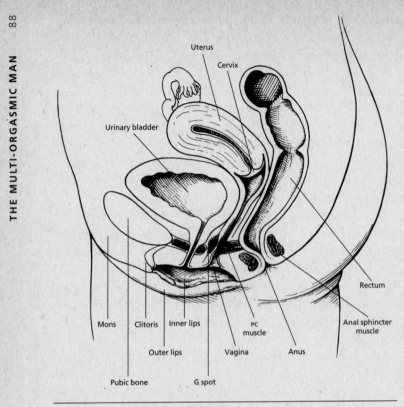

FIGURE 18. WOMAN'S SEXUAL ANATOMY

opposed to men's largely external) sex organs have made them the subject of much study and even more confusion. Every man (and woman) needs to know a few basic facts about women's bodies (see figure 18). Bear in mind that these are generic descriptions and that sexual anatomy, women's and men's, varies as much from person to person as does the rest of our anatomy.

MONS VENERIS

Descending down from a woman's belly, you will first see her mons veneris, which in Latin means "mount of Venus." Venus, of course, was the goddess of love. The mons (for short) is the layer of padded, generally hair-covered skin on top of the pubic bone. As a teenager you probably felt this part of your girlfriend's body if you ever "bumped and grinded" with your clothes on. The mons is just above the clitoris; some women find this area to be sensitive to touch and pressure, while others will want you to focus farther down.

OUTER LIPS

The mons as it descends between a woman's thighs separates into two large outer lips. Although these are called "lips," when a woman is not aroused they are relatively flat and don't look very liplike.

INNER LIPS

Unlike the outer lips, the inner lips are hairless and are related to other mucous membranes like the lips of the mouth. When unaroused, they vary in color from pink to maroon or purple. During sexual arousal, they become engorged, darken, and thicken. They can sometimes swell as much as two to three times their normal size and change in color to bright red. These changes are also a sign of great arousal and approaching orgasm.

CLITORIS

Follow the inner lips up to where they meet just below the mons. There they form the hood that protects the sensitive glans of the clitoris, which is similar to the glans (head) of a man's penis in its abundance of sensitive nerves. Usually the glans is nestled under the hood, but it can be seen by pulling the hood gently back. The glans is so sensitive that quite a few women find direct stimulation painful. These women often prefer stimulation of the shaft of the clitoris, which stretches up toward the mons and can be felt under the skin as a movable cord. After orgasm, many women find that their clitoris is too sensitive to be touched directly for up to several minutes. This hypersensitivity is similar to what many men experience after ejaculating.

Like the penis, the clitoris is made of erectile tissue, and the glans engorges with blood when excited. Many people compare the clitoris to the head of the penis, and developmentally they originate from the same embryonic tissue. The clitoris, however, is unique in being the only organ in either sex that exists exclusively for sexual pleasure. So much for the belief that women are less lusty than men: they are the ones who have a part of their body wholly dedicated to getting them hot and bothered.

URETHRA

Down from the clitoris is the opening to the urethra, which leads to the bladder. Unlike men, whose urethra is relatively long (extending through their penis), women have a relatively short tube to the bladder, which is a major reason women tend to get more urinary-tract and bladder infections than men. The in-out thrusting of intercourse can push bacteria up a woman's urethra. If your partner gets infections frequently, encourage her to urinate after lovemaking. This will help flush out bacteria.

VAGINA

Down from the clitoris and urethra is the entrance to the vagina. The walls of the vagina rest against one another, creating a potential space rather than an actual one. The walls of the vagina have many folds, which explains the vagina's ability to accommodate almost any size penis, not to mention a baby during childbirth. This ability to expand and contract, even to fit snugly around a finger, is the reason differences in penis size are not usually a problem.

At rest, the back wall of the vagina is about three inches long and the front wall is about two and a half inches long. As a woman is aroused, her vagina widens and lengthens. The inner two-thirds of the vagina balloons out, which often reduces the stimulation in the back, but the outer third actually tightens as it becomes engorged, which is one reason a woman can hold on to even a small penis. As we mentioned in the last chapter, the stronger your partner's PC muscles, the more she can contract her vagina around your penis and increase stimulation for both of you. If your partner enjoys deep penetration and you have difficulty stimulating the back of her vagina, especially once it has expanded, you will be pleased to hear that there are positions that shorten her vagina and make deep thrusting easier (see the section called "Positions for Pleasure and Health" in the next chapter).

Many women report that they are most sensitive near the opening of the vagina, but other women report sensitivity at other places throughout the vagina, including the back walls and even the cervix (see the following section, "The G Spot and Other Sensitive Spots"). There are no universals about sexual stimulation, even with the best efforts of researchers like Masters and Johnson to find them. So explore with your partner, and let her tell you what feels best.

THE G SPOT AND OTHER SENSITIVE SPOTS

You may have heard about a place in a woman's vagina that when touched can drive her wild. This spot is often called the G spot, named for physician Ernest Gräfenberg, who first described it in 1950. Although not new, the idea of the G spot is still controversial, some women finding it and others not. The current theory is that the G spot is a collection of glands, ducts, blood vessels, and nerve endings that surround a woman's urethra.

So where exactly is it? Most women who report finding the G spot locate it one and a half to two inches from the opening of the vagina on the upper front wall, just behind the pubic bone. (Some women, however, find their G spot farther back.) If you look at your partner's vagina and imagine a clock with the clitoris as twelve o'clock, the G spot is usually somewhere between eleven and one.

When a woman is not aroused, the G spot is more difficult to find, but you may be able to feel some bumpy or ridged skin. When stimulated it can swell to the size of a dime or larger, standing out from the wall of the vagina. Alan and Donna Brauer suggest that the best time to find it is just after a woman orgasms: "It is already somewhat enlarged and sensitive." They recommend stroking it at a rate of about once a second and experimenting with both lighter and heavier pressure. Another good time to stimulate the G spot is when your partner is just approaching orgasm. Either way, your partner is more likely to enjoy this stroking if you do it once she is already highly aroused. Try licking her clitoris with your tongue while touching her G spot with your finger and see how she responds!

You should know that some women feel initial discomfort or the urge to urinate when their G spot is stroked, so you should probably discuss your exploratory plans with your partner first and explain that this reaction, if it happens, is normal. The Brauers also suggest lightening your touch. It may take as much as a minute for the discomfort or seeming need to urinate to be replaced with pleasurable sensations. If she is uncomfortable or too concerned about urinating to enjoy your stroking, you might suggest that she try to find the G spot on her own at first. It is easiest for her to find it while sitting or squatting. (If she is concerned about feeling the need to urinate, have your partner sit on the toilet or urinate before lovemaking, which will convince her that her bladder is empty.)

Intercourse in the common face-to-face "missionary" position often misses the G spot completely. It is easier to stimulate this area with your penis if your partner lies on her stomach and you enter her from behind, or if she is on top, where she can position herself for her pleasure. Shallow thrusting is also best for stimulating her G spot. Fingers, however, are usually the most direct and effective way to stimulate her G spot at first.

Some women report that their most sensitive spots are located at the four o'clock and eight o'clock positions, about midway back along the walls of the vagina. There are nerve bundles at these locations, which may explain their sensitivity to pressure. Through stroking her vagina or thrusting in different directions, you may already have discovered that your partner has additional spots all her own.

Remember, though, that not all women have a G spot or any other particular "spot," and if your partner doesn't, the last thing you want to do is pressure her or make her feel inadequate. This whole exploration is for her pleasure and is not an attempt to find buttons or knobs that turn her on. Make G-spot stimulation a part of the smorgasbord of pleasure you offer her.

EJACULATION

Female ejaculation? A number of sexologists have in fact described the G spot's ability to "ejaculate" a clear liquid when highly aroused. This has led some to conclude that the G spot may be analogous to a man's prostate gland. (As we mentioned earlier, men's and women's sex organs develop out of the same tissue in the embryo.) Many women who ejaculate worry that they are urinating and, as we mentioned above, may feel an initial need to urinate when their G spot is touched. However, the liquid is definitely not urine, and the urge to urinate usually subsides quickly with increased arousal.

You may at some point feel a "spray" against your penis when making love. Occasionally this spray is even visible. A small number of women ejaculate a teaspoon or less of liquid out of their urethra when they orgasm. (Women who ejaculate should also try to draw their sexual energy up, since they will lose some energy through ejaculating—though less than a man does.) According to researcher Lonnie Barbach, "recent chemical analysis of the [female] ejaculatory fluid suggests that it is unlike either urine or vaginal lubrication, but rather is like male ejaculatory fluid in its high levels of glucose and acid phosphatase. It is believed that the source of the fluid is a system of glands and ducts called the paraurethral glands. These surround the female urethra and develop from the same embryological tissue that develops into the prostate in the male."[2] Explainable or not, this female ejaculate can be quite startling if you are unfamiliar with it. One man described getting hit in the face the first time he went down on his girlfriend. This propulsive force is probably a rare occurrence, but don't be shocked if you find that with some women you need oral-sex goggles.

ANUS

For some women the anus is an erogenous zone, and for others it is off-limits. You should ask how your partner feels. If you and she are interested in anal intercourse or anal sex play (touching and entering her anus with your finger), it is always best to start slowly and sensitively and to make sure you have plenty of lubricant. If her anus constricts while you are stimulating it, you need to apply less stimulation. If her anus is relaxed, you can apply more stimulation.

BREASTS

Compared with the rest of a woman's sexual anatomy, breasts are relatively simple. The nipples rest on top of the dark circles of the areolae and become erect when aroused. For all their erotic significance, the breasts are really quite similar to sweat glands, and their primary role, as any breast-feeding mother will attest, is as a source of warm milk for babies. One could come up with interesting theories as to why in our bottle-fed, nurture-starved Western culture, large breasts have become such a powerful symbol of desire. Whatever the reason is, this flood of images has led many men (and women) to the mistaken belief that size reflects sexual appetite: the larger the breasts, the more sexually desirous a woman is. In actual fact, a woman's sexual sensitivity, experience, and self-perception determine the responsiveness of her breasts, as they do with her sexuality in general. Size has nothing to do with it.

In the "buttons and knobs" view of arousal, men often zero in on their partner's nipples. Though some women enjoy immediate nipple stimulation, many prefer a lighter, more indirect touch to begin with. Generally, try to circle around your partner's breasts to increase her anticipation and desire before actually touching the nipples themselves. Some women, however, experience very little sensation when their breasts or nipples are touched, so don't be disappointed. Rubbing your fingers together to warm them before touching her nipples will increase the amount of *chi,* or energy, and can help stimulate her. As you touch her nipples lightly, you may be able to feel a current of electricity flowing between your finger and her nipple. Licking her nipples with your tongue is often very effective since your tongue has a lot of *chi.* Sometimes, as with many men, the nerve pathways to the nipples need activating, which can occur with gentle, gradual stimulation over time. But your partner needs to be open to this slow awakening.

FERTILITY

The cycles of a woman's fertility and menstruation are especially bewildering for most men and have resulted in much fear and confusion. This is not the place for a biology lesson, but there are a few biological facts that every man should know about his lover's body. For example, did you know that although a woman's egg lives for only twelve to twenty-four hours, she can actually get pregnant as long as five days after intercourse?

How is this possible? Before a woman's ovary releases an egg, her cervical glands release "fertile" mucus. This mucus helps the semen reach the egg, and within ten minutes after ejaculation sperm are already in the fallopian tubes "breathlessly" flapping their tails toward the egg. Other sperm, however, stay in the lining of the cervical canal, where they are nourished and released over a period of three to five days. So if you have intercourse on Saturday night and she has fertile mucus but doesn't ovulate until Tuesday, you could still become a father on Wednesday. (This is a public-service announcement from your local chapter of Planned Parenthood.)

Many women complain that their partners do not take an active role in thinking about, planning, and participating in contraception. With the increased use of condoms, this situation is changing, but not enough. It's good to know the difference between fertile and nonfertile mucus, since condoms do break and no birth control is flawless. Fertile mucus is clear, slick, and stretchy. If you place some between your thumb and forefinger, it will stretch as you sep- arate your fingers, connecting them by a thin, clear thread of mucus. If her mucus is not fertile, it will be white, sticky, and less abundant. Most noticeably, it does not stretch like fertile mucus.

If a woman does not become pregnant, the blood and cells that were prepared to nourish the fertilized egg slough off, beginning her menstruation. The menstrual cycle varies tremendously. Few women have an exact twenty-eight-day cycle. Regular cycles can range from three to seven weeks, and some women menstruate only two or three times a year. Although menstruation is different for every woman, the typical pattern of bleeding starts with a light flow of pink-tinged mucus or drops of blood, increasing to a heavy flow of red blood, and then decreasing to brownish "spotting" be- fore stopping altogether. Some women bleed a lot, others a little, but most stop bleeding within a week.

During menstruation many women experience symptoms such as sore breasts, bloatedness, pimples, headaches, lower-back pain, diarrhea, and constipation. (Women with chronic herpes may break out around this time as well.) As you can imagine, given all of these discomforts, not to mention the stigma that still surrounds men- struation, many women do not feel very sexual during this time. Others, however, find that menstruation is the time of their greatest arousal, and indeed every part of the cycle is experienced by some women as the time of their most intense desire. For a number of women intercourse during menstruation can even relieve cramping. The more you understand about your partner's cycle and the more understanding you can be, the more you can harmonize with her through the rhythmic flow of living as well as the rhythmic flow of lovemaking.

Her Orgasm

The female orgasm has been the source of centuries, if not millennia, of curiosity and controversy, with widespread acceptance by the medical establishment of its existence occurring only in the last hundred years. Even with its existence acknowledged, the female orgasm has endured much ignorance and confusion during this century. The main debate was waged over the differences between, and the relative "maturity" of, clitoral orgasms and vaginal orgasms.[3] We now know that some women have orgasms more easily when their clitoris is stimulated and others have orgasms more easily when their vagina is stimulated. It is as simple as that. The one is no better than the other.

CLITORAL AND VAGINAL ORGASMS

A current theory suggests that there are actually two distinct nerves that are responsible for the two different orgasms. The pudendal nerve goes to the clitoris, among other places, and the pelvic nerve goes to the vagina and uterus—vaginal orgasms often actually involve contractions of the uterus as well (see figure 30 on page 154). Of the two nerves, the pudendal has more nerve endings, which may be the reason more women have clitoral orgasms than have vaginal orgasms. The fact that the two nerves overlap in the spinal cord also might explain why some women have "blended" orgasms, which arise from both the clitoris and deep inside the vagina. Two factors seem to influence whether women have vaginal orgasms: the strength of their PC muscles and the sensitivity of their G spots or other internal spots.

Women who have both orgasms often notice a difference. Shere Hite, in her famous report on female sexuality, quotes a woman who explains her experience: "During masturbation I experience a clitoral orgasm that approximates my idea of male orgasm—a buildup of overall sensation in the general area of my clitoris, and a 'muscle spasm' feeling. A vaginal orgasm is a more pervasive sensation through the whole body, less concrete to describe—wider waves of feeling." As we described in chapter 2, men can be said to have two different orgasms as well: a genital (or penis) orgasm and a pelvic (or prostate) orgasm. According to Taoist sexuality, there are actually numerous kinds of orgasms, which can take place in different parts and, believe it or not, different organs of the body, such as your heart and liver. If you are able to circulate your sexual energy to your brain, you may experience a "brain orgasm." Remember, an orgasm is simply the contraction and expansion, or "pulsation," and this pulsation can happen throughout your entire body.

TOUCHING HER CLITORIS DURING LOVEMAKING

Shere Hite reports that about 70 percent of the women she surveyed required at least some stimulation of their clitoris in order to have an orgasm. As already mentioned, your partner's clitoris is equivalent to the head of your penis. For the majority of men, the head is the most sensitive part of their sexual anatomy—as is the clitoris for most women. Asking a woman to have an orgasm without stimulating her clitoris is like asking a man to have an orgasm without stimulating the head of his penis. It can be done, but it takes a lot longer.

It is not surprising then that in the missionary position many women are not able to have an orgasm, since the most sensitive part of their anatomy—the clitoris—is only indirectly being stimulated. Sometimes the man's pubic bone will rub against the clitoris or the hood of the clitoris will be pulled against it during intercourse, but these are clearly no substitute for direct stimulation by your penis, fingers, or mouth. It's not surprising that Kinsey, Hunt, and Hite have all found that nearly half of American women never or rarely experience orgasm during intercourse.

Many women are much more easily orgasmic during intercourse if they, or their partners, also stimulate their clitoris. Men usually can orgasm much more quickly than women during intercourse

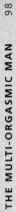

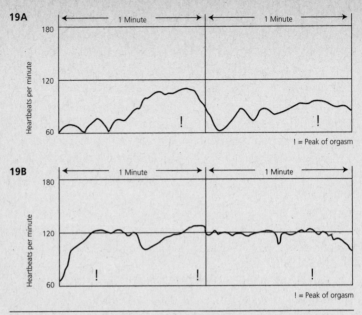

FIGURE 19. DISCRETE (A) AND CONTINUOUS (B) FEMALE MULTIPLE ORGASMS
(Source: Hartman and Fithian)

(two or three minutes versus twenty), but women seem to be able to orgasm just as quickly as men when they masturbate—presumably because they are directly stimulating their clitoris and because they know what they like. One multi-orgasmic man recounted his experience of stroking his partner's clitoris while making love: "When I'm behind or she's on top, my hands are free to play with her clitoris. It really drives her wild. She starts moaning so loud that once we had to stop and close the windows."

Some men and women may complain that using hands to stimulate your partner's clitoris during intercourse is unnatural or overly mechanical. As one multi-orgasmic man remembered, "For a long time I thought it was a sign of weakness for a man to have to use his fingers. But I've found that there are some times when a woman really enjoys or would even rather have your fingers or tongue, because it is a whole different feeling." Surely this kind of stimulation cannot be considered unnatural or a sign of a man's weakness if almost three-quarters of all women require it to be sexually satisfied.

Men who are not used to using their hands when they have intercourse may find that they need a little time to coordinate their strokes and their thrusts. With practice, this coordination becomes increasingly easy, especially if you slow your thrusting down and allow your partner (and yourself) to savor every thrust and every stroke. You need to be careful not to become overly focused on your partner's clitoris and lose the connection of lovemaking. Also be careful not to lose track of what your hand is doing, or your partner may start to feel like it *is* becoming mechanical. If you can walk and chew gum at the same time, you should be able to simultaneously thrust and stroke.

If your partner is willing to touch herself, all the better. One man told his girlfriend that because she was involved in bringing herself to orgasm, he felt like she was using him to "masturbate." This reaction might be understandable if a man feels that it is his responsibility (and his right) to "give" his partner orgasms. This mind-set no doubt underlies women's faking orgasm to please their partners or to show their partners they have been pleased. Since, as we explained in chapter 2, orgasm takes place primarily in the brain, you cannot "give" your partner an orgasm. She must experience it in her own mind (and body).

As more and more women have discovered their ability to orgasm once or multiple times, men have felt increasing pressure to satisfy this ever higher orgasmic potential. Men's desire to satisfy women is noble and necessary, but the accompanying pressure is not and can increase already too common feelings of performance anxiety among men. You will   e a more realistic approach, and feel much less pressure, if you realize that you are simply helping your partner reach her own orgasmic potential.

ORGASMIC FINGERPRINTING

Clitoral, vaginal, and blended orgasms are just three categories that sexologists use to describe genital orgasms in women. As we mentioned in chapter 2, sexologists also make distinctions between brief, *discrete* orgasms and longer, *continuous* orgasms (see figure 19). Some women have discrete orgasms, others have continuous orgasms, and still others have a combination. Hartman, Fithian, and coauthor Berry Campbell suggest that each woman's pattern of orgasm is so individual that it should be called an "orgasmic fingerprint." As Lonnie Barbach has pointed out, physiology as well as personal and cultural expectations influence how your partner (and you) experience orgasm, which is probably one of the reasons people tend to have a "standard" orgasmic pattern. Some women have one powerful orgasm, some have one gentle orgasm, and some have one continuous orgasm. Women who are multi-orgasmic can have any combination of the above. It is important to remember that your partner's orgasm (like your own) will be somewhat different each time.

According to Sexual Kung Fu, women can also direct their energy out of their pelvis and up to their brain, and expand their orgasms throughout their entire body. This circulation of *chi* will energize your partner just as it energizes you. (In chapter 6, we suggest exercises your partner can do to expand her orgasms.) Women in general are less genitally focused than men and, as a result, have an easier time experiencing and expanding their orgasms throughout their bodies. Perhaps as a result of this diffusion, many women are genitally "preorgasmic" (that is, have never had a genital orgasm). In chapter 6, we offer techniques for preorgasmic women to become orgasmic as well as techniques for orgasmic women to become multi-orgasmic.

It will be much easier for you to become a multi-orgasmic man if your partner enjoys long periods of lovemaking. More couples suffer from the man's not being able to last long enough than from the woman's growing tired before the man. However, the latter can be the case if you become multi-orgasmic and she does not. Although it is important not to pressure her and to accept her desires for more or less pleasure, you should encourage her to explore her potential through the chapter written for her. In chapter 9, we also offer suggestions for couples for whom there is a serious imbalance in sexual appetite. Most women, however, will want to help their partners become multi-orgasmic, and the most important thing your partner can do to help is to explore her own pleasure and cultivate her own sexual satisfaction.

Her Arousal

Most women take longer to become aroused than most men, but once women are aroused, their desire can generally outlast that of their partners. (As a Sexual Kung Fu practitioner, you will be an exception to the second part of this rule.) According to Taoism, men are like fire and women are like water. Fire ignites quickly but can easily be quenched by water. To satisfy your lover, you need to bring her desire to a boil, which requires that you keep your fire burning long enough to do so. The secret to satisfying your partner is to understand the stages of her arousal and to learn how to synchronize your arousal with hers.

HOW DO I KNOW WHEN A WOMAN'S DESIRE IS BOILING?

Taoist physicians recorded the stages of arousal they noticed in women. Many of their observations have been confirmed by Western research, especially by Kinsey in a chapter of his *Sexual Behavior in the Human Female* entitled "Physiology of Sexual Response and Orgasm." We note the stages here not to make women feel self-conscious but to help men understand how to better satisfy their partner's desires. As you are reading about these general stages, it is important to keep in mind Kinsey's conclusion about the uniqueness of each person's sexuality: "There is nothing more characteristic of the sexual response than the fact that it is not the same in any two individuals."

With this said, we could not have a better guide to a general description of women's arousal than Su Nü, one of the Yellow Emperor's trusted female advisers. The Yellow Emperor once asked her, "How can I tell if the woman is experiencing pleasure?" Su Nü replied that there are Five Signs, Five Desires, and Ten Movements that demonstrate a woman's growing arousal. The Five Signs and Five Desires describe what happens to a woman's body as she becomes aroused, while the Ten Movements describe how her actions convey what she wants you to do next.

Before describing these secrets of women's arousal, it is worth mentioning that we live in more open and direct times than did Su

Nü, and you do not have to limit yourself to reading the tea leaves of your partner's body. You can also ask her what she wants; better still, she may tell you. However, the throes of lovemaking are not always conducive to speech, let alone a clear statement of preferences. Passion overwhelms language, and it is at this time that it will help if you have learned to recognize a woman's mounting pleasure. Before or after lovemaking, you can discuss with your partner whether Su Nü understood her individual desires. It should go without saying that consent is essential in any sexual encounter, and the fact that you notice that the body of the woman you are dating is becoming aroused means nothing unless her mind wants to act on it. "No" means no, regardless of what her body says.

The Taoist texts were at times extremely direct and at other times quite vague. Some of the stages of arousal will seem clear, even obvious, while others may seem too subtle to detect. The Signs, Desires, and Movements overlap somewhat and are difficult to keep straight, so we will try to simplify them below. Remember that these are general signposts and not an exact road map. Don't expect to notice each stage each time you make love, and do not wait to check off each one before proceeding. Above all, lovemaking should be fluid and spontaneous, and these signposts will simply help you stay on the right course.

THE SIGNS OF DESIRE

As ejaculatory control begins with breathing, so too does passion, and the first signal you will have of your lover's desire is a change in her breathing, which will become increasingly rapid and shallow. According to Su Nü, if her nostrils flare and her mouth widens and she embraces you with both arms, she wants your and her genitals to touch. When her body quivers, she wants you to touch her genitals gently. If her face becomes flushed, she wants you to play with the head of your penis around her mons, and when she stretches out her legs, she wants you to rub the head of your penis against her clitoris and the entrance to her vagina.

Su Nü continues: If her nipples harden and she pushes out her belly, slowly and shallowly enter her. If her throat is dry and she swallows saliva, slowly begin to move inside her. If she starts to move her bottom, she is experiencing great pleasure. If her vagina is well lubricated or if she raises her legs to encircle you, enter her more deeply. If she presses her thighs together, her pleasure is becoming overwhelming. If she moves from side to side, she wants you to thrust deeply from side to side. If she is perspiring enough to dampen the sheets or she straightens her body and closes her eyes, she wants to orgasm. If she arches her body against yours, her pleasure has peaked. If she stretches out and relaxes, pleasure fills her entire body. If her vaginal secretions spread down her thighs and over her buttocks, she is fully satisfied and you should slowly withdraw.

Now that we have discussed what signs to *recognize* in your partner's mounting desire, we must discuss how to *satisfy* that desire, which we do in the following chapter.

CHAPTER FIVE

Becoming a Multi-Orgasmic Couple

Controlling your ejaculation while self-pleasuring is one thing, but controlling it during the throes of lovemaking is quite another. The control you developed in chapter 3 over your breathing, your concentration, your PC muscles, and, most important, your sexual energy will help you immeasurably in becoming multi-orgasmic with your partner, but you also need to know the duo practice for lovemaking.

Pleasuring Your Partner

Unlike men's arousal, women's has no precipice. True, many women will have orgasms that they find so fully satisfying (and climactic) that they do not need to continue making love. And as we discussed earlier, some women even ejaculate. But since women do not have to worry about losing an erection or spilling their seed, they can generally surrender themselves to pleasure in a way that men cannot. Nevertheless, women do not fall into bliss without effort. Reaching orgasm, multiple orgasms, and expanded orgasms requires knowledge, skill, and effort of women just as it does of men. Here's how you can help.

In Sexual Kung Fu all aspects of touch are seen as part of the union between man and woman. Touching hands or lips is as much a part of harmonizing with one another as is intercourse. As with self-pleasuring, you probably have your own way of pleasuring your partner, and though most women have the same general erogenous zones, each woman, of course, has different sensitivities at different times. Try out these Taoist techniques, but let your partner's preferences be your guide.

"The essence of foreplay is slowness," states the *Discourse on the Highest Tao Under Heaven*. "If one proceeds slowly and patiently, the woman will be exceedingly joyful. She will adore you like a brother and love you like a parent. One who has mastered this Tao deserves to be called a heavenly gentleman." Because anticipation and growing intensity are important in bringing your partner's desire to a boil, you should begin with passionate kissing. Begin at her extremities rather than her genitals. Caress, massage, and kiss her hands and wrists as well as her feet and ankles. Move up her arms and legs to her abdomen. Stimulating points along the meridians of her body (energy channels) will help increase her sexual excitement: there are many points along or near her spine (the Back Channel), such as the small of her back, her neck, and her ears. The underside of the arms and the inside of the thighs are also very sensitive on most women. By *caress*, we mean that your touch should generally be featherweight, although it can be heavier when you are stimulating larger muscles such as her buttocks.

HER BREASTS

As we mentioned earlier, when you approach her breasts, spiral around them in ever narrower circles until you slowly reach her nipples. Most men go for the nipples too soon. (Old breast-feeding instincts, perhaps.) Circling them slowly will draw her sexual energy to her nipples. Also, remember to rub your thumbs and forefingers together to generate more *chi*. Finally, touch her nipples lightly, and try rolling them between your thumbs and index fingers. (You can touch both breasts or just focus on one at a time.) Some women enjoy harder squeezing and fondling, but let your partner's responses guide you. As we already mentioned, your tongue is highly charged with *chi,* and using it to lick, spiral around, and suck on her nipple is often an excellent way to arouse her. If her nipples become engorged and erect, you are doing something right.

HER GENITALS

In approaching your partner's genitals, it is best to stimulate her inner thighs, mons, and vaginal lips before approaching the clitoris. Imagine that you are moving through concentric circles of increasing pleasure and intensity. When you finally approach her clitoris, her sexual energy and excitement will be enormous.

Each woman likes to have her clitoris touched differently, and you need to become the expert in her particular pleasure. Even more important than where to touch is how to touch. Using your finger, stroke or spiral evenly—not too fast, not too slow. Avoid big movements: the clitoris's sensitivity is far more concentrated than that of the penis, and you are better off with more focused, subtler movements than with the kind of vigorous stimulation that most men enjoy.

As for where to touch, you are best off starting with the less sensitive parts of this very sensitive sex organ. Try stroking the base and sides of the clitoris. Then try stroking the hood and rolling the clitoris between your thumb and index finger—gently! Remember to touch the hood first, before touching the extremely sensitive glans. Experiment with different strokes and varying degrees of pressure. If your partner likes it, she will push her genitals slightly toward you for more stimulation. Moans, sighs, pants, jerking muscles, curling toes, and sweat, as well as smiles and other facial expressions, are all good signs. If your touch is too heavy or uncomfortable, she will pull her pelvis slightly away. Lighten up or try another stroke.

TONGUE KUNG FU

Although effective, fingers are not ideal, because they are not nearly as sensitive as your partner's clitoris. The hardness of the bones in your fingers and the sharpness of your nails can be painful. (Always make sure your nails are short and smooth.) For this reason, your tongue is much better suited to the task.

There have been many jokes about oral sex and its attendant smells and tastes. There are men who grimace at the thought and men who smile with fond memories. One multi-orgasmic man described his conversion to an oral-sex fan: "In the past, I definitely didn't like to use my tongue because it felt like I wasn't getting anything out of it. I was kind of selfish, really—I was a getter. And now my partner will be having these incredible orgasms because of what I am doing with my tongue, and it feels great to watch. I even start tingling in my body. It's true what the Tao says about when you are in tune. I get by giving. This is something a lot of guys miss. I know I did for a long time." Whatever your personal feelings are about oral sex, you should know that it is probably the fastest way to get a woman's vaginal juices flowing in preparation for lovemaking. As we discussed earlier, it is also the easiest, and for some women the only, way in which they have an orgasm.

If you are not a cunnilingus fan, you do not have to dive in headfirst. If you use your tongue on your partner's clitoris, your nose and face will be nearest her mons and lower abdomen. If it is the odor that you object to, you and she can try bathing together or using scented oils. (We should mention that many men are turned on by, or over time come to be turned on by, the smell of their partner's vagina.) Best, of course, is not to focus initially or exclusively on her clitoris: use your tongue to touch her inner lips, the sensitive spot at the base of her vagina, and her perineum as well.

It is also important not to get overly fixated on her genitals to the exclusion of the rest of her body. Some women feel disconnected during oral sex, and this feeling can be lessened by using your hands to continue caressing her legs, belly, breasts, hands, and face. Many women find that having their nipples stimulated during oral sex can heighten their pleasure immensely. Other women find that this distracts them from the intensity of clitoral stimulation. As for clitoral techniques, you probably will want to try a combination of brushing with your lips, flicking with your tongue, and sucking with your mouth. Alternating between using your tongue and gently sucking her clitoris into your mouth can be extremely pleasurable. Again, be careful of too much pressure. Light, consistent, and rhythmic pressure is generally best.

Many men mistakenly think that oral sex involves inserting their tongue into their partner's vagina. This is not generally the case, since the tongue is usually too short and too soft to stimulate a woman's vagina successfully, although Taoists do recommend a technique for stimulating the G spot by hooking your tongue and pulling back. It's worth a try—especially if you have a strong tongue! (You actually can strengthen your tongue by sticking it out and then pulling it in like a snake as fast as you can for a minute or two. Practice as often as you can.)

ENTERING HER

Generally, your fingers are more effective than your tongue for stimulating the inside of your partner's vagina. You can use one finger (or, if she's very aroused, two fingers) to enter her. Circle around the wall of her vagina to find where she is most sensitive. Don't forget to try the G spot about an inch or two behind her clitoris. You may also wish to thrust your fingers in and out (slowly at first), simulating the action of your penis.

At this point, your partner's desire is probably close to boiling and she is eager for you to enter her. But do not enter her quite yet. Hold your penis in your hand as if you were about to guide it into her vagina. But before entering, rub the head of your penis against her clitoris. This will help bring her passion to a rapid boil. Then enter her gradually, first about an inch, then two, and then pull back a little so that your penis is just inside the entrance to her vagina. This slow, lingering approach will help you control your own desire and will allow you to begin a thrusting pattern, which will bring both of you to the peak of pleasure many times.

If she is multi-orgasmic, you may want to help bring her to orgasm before you enter her, or you may want to wait until you have entered her. If she has already orgasmed at least once, she may be more patient with your need to stop momentarily during lovemaking as you approach the point of no return. Also, when you are making love her orgasms actually will help you control your ejaculation. As the Taoists understand it, water (vaginal fluid) cools down fire. As you gain greater mastery over your urge to ejaculate, this will be less of a concern because you will be able to use your breath and your mind more effectively to control this urge and will need to interrupt the rhythm of lovemaking less often.

CHARGING HER EROTIC CIRCUITS

While pleasuring your partner, you should try to avoid sexual scripts or patterns of lovemaking that can become routine. The sequence for pleasuring your partner described in the previous section is not the only one. It generally follows the pattern of arousal for most women, but not necessarily all women and certainly not at all times. During a "quickie," for example, you might want to jump right to oral sex. Mix and match. See what your partner wants and what the mood of the moment is. Although techniques can help you satisfy your partner, it is worth bearing in mind Herant Katchadourian's advice in his *Fundamentals of Human Sexuality:* "A simplistic search for bodily levers and push-buttons leads to mechanical sex since the energy that charges the erotic circuits is emotion." Knowledge of your partner's body is essential, but there is no substitute for sincere affection.

Thrusting Techniques

Most porn movies portray men thrusting in and out, sawing away until they ejaculate. It is no surprise that this is therefore what most men think they should do. In fact, this thrusting rhythm is a recipe for fast ejaculation and little satisfaction for either the man or the woman. The Taoists recognized that proper thrusting was essential for coital pleasure, ejaculatory control, and sexual health. Yet even more important than any particular technique is making sure your partner is already highly aroused. Thrusting in too soon (before she is highly lubricated) should be avoided at all costs. Even if she is eager for you to enter her, a slow hand and pelvis will raise her anticipation and help you control your ejaculation.

FINDING YOUR RHYTHM

The Taoists developed numerous different thrusting patterns, most of which involved varying between shallow thrusts and deep thrusts (see figure 20). All of these patterns encouraged the man to

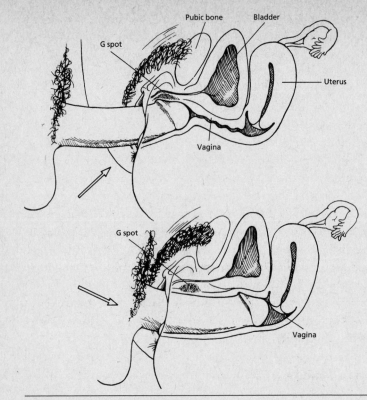

FIGURE 20. SHALLOW AND DEEP THRUSTS

thrust shallowly a number of times before thrusting deeply, the most common involving *nine shallow and one deep*. (As you learn to control your ejaculation, you can lessen the ratio to six or even three shallow to one deep.)

Alternating between shallow and deep thrusts will not only help you last longer; it will also thrill your partner. The deep thrust pushes all of the air out of her vagina, creating a vacuum, which the shallow thrusts intensify. You want to avoid withdrawing completely, which breaks the seal of the vacuum; instead, pull back so that you are about an inch or so inside her. One multi-orgasmic man described his experience: "When I read about this Taoist thrusting technique I really didn't believe it would work, but women just go crazy: they *love* the shallow and deep. They orgasm a lot quicker and can have two or three before I get to one. In the past, I couldn't last long enough to get a woman to that point."

More important than any particular number of shallow and deep thrusts is practicing a basic rhythm that you can maintain and that both you and your partner can enjoy for prolonged periods of time. Don't allow your thrusting to become mechanical by getting lost in counting off numbers.

DEEP THRUSTS

When most men thrust deeply, they pull back all the way, which rubs the head of their penis—their most sensitive spot—against the full length of their partner's vagina. If you have difficulty getting or maintaining an erection, this in-out deep thrust is especially valuable (see the Soft Entry exercise in chapter 8). However, as you can imagine, this thrust is also highly arousing and ordinarily leads to quick ejaculation.

For this reason, the Taoist masters developed the up-down deep thrust. This thrust uses the base of your penis, which is your least sensitive spot, to stimulate your partner's clitoris, which is her most sensitive spot (see figure 21). The benefits for postponing ejaculation are obvious. Instead of pulling back, you can stay deep inside your partner and thrust up and down repeatedly. This is especially important when she is in the midst of orgasming and wants you deep inside her but you are close to the edge.

Keep in mind that women's clitorises differ in their proximity to the vagina, which may be one reason that some women are more easily orgasmic during intercourse than others. You will be able to stimulate some women clitorally just by using the up-down deep thrust, while others will need the help of your fingers. Either way, this thrust will help you immeasurably during the most intense throes of lovemaking.

DIFFERENT DIRECTIONS

In addition to depth, you can also vary the direction in which you thrust. According to Chinese medicine, the parts of the vagina, like the parts of the penis, correspond to the organs and glands of the body (see figure 22). To truly satisfy and energize your partner,

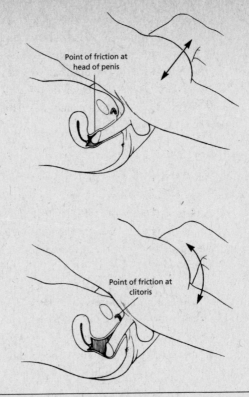

FIGURE 21. IN-OUT THRUST VS. UP-DOWN THRUST

you will need to stimulate her entire vagina during lovemaking. This may seem like a lot of work, and you will not be able to do it every time you make love, but the more of her vagina you can massage with your penis, the better.

Begin by thrusting shallow—left and right, top and bottom. Then thrust deep and, while staying deep, use the base of your shaft to rub up and down against your partner's clitoris and the head of your penis to rub gently against her cervix. Now pull back at an angle, which stimulates the walls of her vagina. (Once you have learned to differentiate between shallow and deep, you can also explore the middle depth.) Remember, women have different spots of greatest sensitivity, so thrusting in different directions has the greatest chance of satisfying your partner.

In addition to depth and direction, you can also vary the speed at which you thrust. The seventh-century physician Li Tung-hsüan Tzu waxed poetic about nine different kinds of thrusts that offer your partner a range of depths, directions, and speeds:

1. Strike left and right as a brave general breaking through the enemy's ranks. [The battle-of-the-sexes imagery was not completely absent from Taoist sexuality.]

2. Rise and suddenly plunge like a wild horse bucking through a mountain stream.

3. Push in and pull out like a flock of seagulls playing on the waves.

4. Use deep thrusts and shallow teasing strokes, like a sparrow plucking pieces of rice.

5. Make shallow and then deeper thrusts in steady succession [to the left and right], like a large stone sinking into the sea.

6. Push in slowly as a snake entering its hole.

7. Charge quickly like a frightened mouse running into its hole.

8. Hover and then strike like an eagle catching an elusive hare.

9. Rise up and then plunge down low like a great sailboat in a wild wind.

In the end you will put the various thrusts you have learned together in your own special pelvic rhythm depending on the time and place—and the pleasure desired.

The Advanced Art of Screwing

When most men thrust, they stimulate only a small part of their partner's entire vagina. This is why advanced Sexual Kung Fu involves "screwing" rather than "thrusting." Although the word *screw* has come to have vulgar connotations in our culture, it is actually quite accurate to describe the spiraling action the Tao suggests for truly pleasuring your partner (and yourself). Instead of thrusting forward and pulling back, you should "screw" your hips or ideally

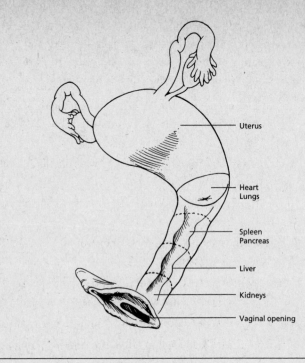

Uterus

Heart
Lungs

Spleen
Pancreas

Liver

Kidneys

Vaginal opening

FIGURE 22.   REFLEXOLOGY POINTS OF THE VAGINA

your sacrum in half circles, first on one side and then the other. One multi-orgasmic man explained his technique: "I will go in circling and come out circling. Play with one side and then play with the other side. I go shallow and then I go deeper, playing with one side and then the other. And then I do a lot more circles. And I've found that a lot of women really love this, especially when having their later orgasms."

More experienced lovers the world over have discovered the effectiveness of moving their hips during lovemaking, and many men find that rocking their shoulders initially helps them to rotate their sacrum or their hips. Your hips, however, are not nearly as subtle and effective as your sacrum, which sits at the center of the pelvis (see figure 23). According to the Tao, it is the sacrum that controls the penis.

Rotating Your Sacrum

At first your rotations will probably come from your hips or pelvis, since, unless you do a lot of Latin or African dance, you are probably not used to rotating your sacrum. Give it time, but eventually you will be able to spiral, to "screw," with subtle movements of your sacrum. To isolate your sacrum, put one hand on your pubis and one hand on your sacrum and try to spiral left and then right. Next, try tilting your penis up as you push your tailbone (the base of your sacrum) forward (curving your back out slightly), and then try tilting your penis down as you push your tailbone back (arching your spine slightly). Once you have isolated your sacrum, you can really screw.

According to the Tao, a nail (thrusting straight in) comes out easily, but a screw (circling) stays in a long time. Elvis Presley used these pelvic (actually, sacral) gyrations onstage to great effect and great popularity, and you will find that you are met with similar applause in the bedroom once you master this technique.

There is even a time and a place for the old bedspring-squeaking hard thrusting, especially if your partner likes very deep penetration and you have a lot of control. One multi-orgasmic man explained: "Women usually like the hard thrusting later on after they are relaxed. If it's too soon, it can be a bit painful. So as the night goes on I find myself thrusting harder because their passion is ready for it. If it gets to be too much for me, I really need to breathe and if absolutely necessary sometimes to pull out and use my tongue and fingers." One of the benefits of using a condom—one that we discuss in the section called "When to Start: A Few Words About Safer Sex" later in this chapter—is that by desensitizing your penis you can make your lovemaking last longer, especially if your partner wants you to

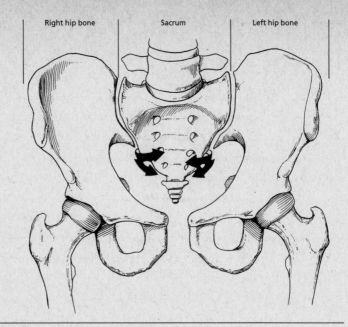

FIGURE 23. ROTATING YOUR SACRUM

thrust hard and deep. But you need to make sure you stay connected to your groin and monitor your rising arousal rate.

The more you practice, the more control you will develop and the less you will need to pull out. One multi-orgasmic man explained what he does when he approaches the point of no return: "When I am making love and start feeling like I am going to come, I really try to listen to my body, and share with my partner where I am and how close I am getting. And if I get real close, I'll stop and do the deep breathing, which will get my body to relax."

You are almost always better off starting with slow thrusts or spirals. (The Taoist practice is the opposite of the hurried, short, and selfish sentiment expressed in the popular description of male sexuality "Wham, bam, thank you, ma'am.") Like all physical and spiritual practices, lovemaking requires both discipline and innovation. You are interested in both: a general pattern of pleasurable thrusting/screwing and a variety of spontaneous changes in depth, speed, and direction.

The Big Draw for Two

We introduced the Big Draw technique in chapter 3 but will discuss it here for you to practice with your partner. In the Big Draw during lovemaking, you will both be trying to multiply and expand your orgasms within yourselves. In the Soul-Mating exercise described later in this chapter, you will also learn to exchange sexual energy with your partner, but for now simply learn to circulate your sexual energy within your own body.

We have divided this practice into its sequential stages so that you can learn it more easily, but when you use it with your partner, it should blend together into a fluid and graceful experience.

It may seem difficult at first to stop yourself from ejaculating given all the pleasurable sensations and expansive desire you feel with your partner. You should keep in mind that you are training your body in this practice and that each time you succeed it becomes easier the next time.

The time between when you start to experience arousal and when an orgasm is imminent is the time you should draw the energy up. If you wait too long, you may not be able to stop it from pouring out. As you become able to separate orgasm from ejaculation, you can draw the energy up as you are experiencing the contractile-phase genital contractions, expanding the orgasm throughout your body.

If you have trouble drawing the energy up to your head, first draw it up to your tailbone and feel it entering your sacrum and the point on your spine opposite your navel from where you can pour the energy into the navel. Once it has pooled there, try to draw it the rest of the way to your head.

TALKING WITH YOUR PARTNER

At first the Sexual Kung Fu practice may seem a little awkward and an interruption in your lovemaking, but it will quickly become increasingly natural and part of a less frenetic, but much more meaningful and pleasurable, style of lovemaking. However, in the meantime it will require support and patience from your partner, which is why it is important to explain to your partner what you are

THE BIG DRAW DURING LOVEMAKING

EMBRACE When you are both highly aroused, stop and hold each other. Look deeply into each other's eyes. Truly see your partner's inner goodness, and express the depth of your love for her with your eyes. Keeping your eyes open also helps bring the energy up. Send each other energy through your gaze, your lips, the palms of your hands, and the surface of your skin.

THRUST/SCREW When your partner is highly aroused, use the head of your penis to rub her inner vaginal lips and especially her clitoris. When she is ready, you will be able to tell by her swollen lips and clitoris and the abundance of her vaginal juices. Enter your partner slowly. You may want to start with a pattern of nine shallow thrusts and one deep thrust. (Remember, these are general guidelines, not rules.)

CONTRACT While still inside your partner, lightly contract the head and base of your penis and your PC muscle. You will be using your mind as well as your pelvic muscles to squeeze these "round" muscles. If necessary, use your fingers to squeeze the base of your penis.

PAUSE When you feel you are near orgasm, pull back so that only about an inch or two of your penis (the head, mostly) is inside your partner's vagina. Make sure you communicate to your partner that you are close to the edge and that she needs to avoid pushing you over the edge. (Pull out all the way only if absolutely necessary.)

DRAW Squeeze your anus and use your mind to draw the energy up from the tip of your penis, through your perineum and tailbone, and up your spine to your head (see the Cool Draw and the Big Draw in chapter 3). This will help spread the orgasmic energy from your genitals, decreasing the urge to ejaculate while expanding your orgasm from a genital orgasm to a whole-body orgasm.

RELAX Relaxing allows the blood vessels in your penis to dilate and allows you to exchange more of your sexual energy with your partner. Your erection may decrease somewhat, which will let the hormone-filled blood return to fortify the rest of your body and allow new blood to flow into your penis when you get hard again. Continue holding each other, kissing, and circulating energy. When ready, you can continue thrusting/screwing and repeat the Big Draw until both of you are completely satisfied.

doing. One multi-orgasmic man remembered: "My girlfriend responded in a very open and positive way. Her reaction was certainly influenced by the fact that our sex quickly became more beautiful. It was also quite important that I practiced often by myself so I rarely had to interrupt our lovemaking to control ejaculation. Of course, it was certainly necessary to explain to my partner what I was doing so she could understand the process."

You can encourage your partner to read chapter 6, but if timing and passion do not afford you this opportunity, you will want to tell her in a few breathless words what you are doing. One multi-orgasmic man described how he explains his practice: "I tell the woman I am with that my sexual philosophy now is this Taoist philosophy. And I ask her for help. Usually I wait until after we've been in bed for a while, and I'll say, 'There's going to come a time where I may need you to help me to stop. You know, I might need to withdraw, I might need to have a little bit of slowing down.' So I let them know why I might want to do that, and what my thinking is. I find that women really respect it and they love hearing about it and it is exciting to them."

It is essential that you tell your partner enough so that she can support your practice. As one multi-orgasmic man explained, "When I am really starting to feel my pumpers wanting to start to pump, I have to slow down more often and sort of just breathe and do the practice. And that's when I start explaining to them what I am doing and why I am doing it, why it is important to me and I think it is important to both of us. Before I explain what I am doing, a lot of women, when I say I am about to come, will say, 'Well, come, come. I like it when you come.' That's when I say, 'I really appreciate that you want to do that for me, but I don't want to come because I don't want to fall asleep right away. I want to have fun. I want to keep my energy up.' And they just understand why, every once in a while, I will need to pull back and take some deep breaths."

Positions for Pleasure and Health

The Taoists were highly inventive in coming up with new and interesting sexual positions. However, for the Taoists these positions

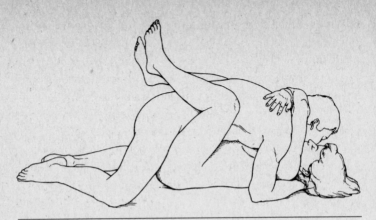

FIGURE 24. MAN-ON-TOP POSITION

were not just for variety; each had a different energetic and healing function. They believed that love expressed through sexuality was the most potent medicine, and a Taoist physician might prescribe several weeks of dedicated lovemaking in a specific position for a particular ailment. If you want to explore these various positions with your partner and use them for self-healing, they are described in *Healing Love Through the Tao: Cultivating Female Sexual Energy* (see appendix). Here we will give the basic and most important positions, as well as some general advice for whatever position you choose. These positions can help enormously in accommodating different body sizes and genital sizes, as well as stimulating different sexual sensitivities. As you and your partner refine your understanding of your sexual pleasures, you will be able to select positions that match these preferences.

FINDING THE WAY

Basic Guidelines

Before we discuss specific positions, there are two basic guidelines that will help you select the correct position for the mood and moment.

1. For relaxing and harmonizing with your partner, place similar body parts together: lips to lips, hands to

hands, genitals to genitals. For stimulating and exciting one another, place dissimilar body parts together: lips to ear, mouth to genitals, genitals to anus.

2. The person who moves (generally the person on top) gives the most energy to the other partner. The person underneath can move as well to complement the movement of the person on top. This will help expand, circulate, and exchange the *chi* more quickly. In the West we assume that the person on top is dominant. How different is the Taoist understanding that the person on top is actually serving the other by sending the most healing energy to him or her. Passion and health, not power, are the main concerns of the skilled Taoist.[1] Your lovemaking should observe these guidelines so that you and your partner both harmonize and excite, heal and are healed.

MAN ON TOP

Even before missionaries made their way to China, the Taoists were well acquainted with the position in which the man lies on top of the woman, usually supporting himself on his hands or elbows. One of the primary benefits of this position is that you and your partner can gaze into each other's eyes and kiss passionately. The face-to-face position is deeply satisfying to your emotions and sense organs, all five of which (eyes, tongue, ear, nose, and skin) come into direct contact. These organs, especially your tongue and eyes, are major carriers of life-force energy (see "Sexing the Spirit" later in this chapter).

In this position your partner can run her hand along your spine to help you draw your energy up to your head. Also in this position many parts of your body—legs, belly, chest, and so on—are in contact with hers, and your weight on your partner's pubic bone and breasts can help her become aroused quickly. This position also allows you to use your thrusting and screwing techniques, both to satisfy your partner and to maintain control of your arousal.

The main drawbacks of the position are that your hands are usually involved in holding yourself up and that your partner's G spot is bypassed almost entirely unless you tilt your sacrum and angle your penis up. You can address this problem by having your partner place a pillow under her buttocks so that her pelvis is tilted back. She can also drape her legs over your arms or shoulders, which has the same effect as the pillow and also allows you to penetrate more deeply. The higher her legs, the deeper the penetration. This is especially helpful if your partner has a relatively large vagina and you have a relatively small penis.

Remember that according to Taoism, man is like fire and woman is like water. Since women take longer to boil, it is often good for the man to begin on top. When the woman's desire is boiling and risks quenching the man's fire (causing him to ejaculate), you may wish to switch to the woman-on-top position, which allows the man to concentrate more easily. In this position, however, the woman must be willing to stop as the man draws close to the point of no return.

WOMAN ON TOP

In this position, the man lies on his back and the woman straddles him. Most men find that this is the easiest position in which to learn to control their ejaculations and to become multi-orgasmic. The reason for this is that you can relax your pelvic muscles in this position and pay close attention to your arousal rate. Gravity also assists in ejaculatory control, and the man can focus on directing the energy up his spine.

Your partner, in this position, can also direct your penis to the most sensitive places in her vagina, including her G spot, which is one reason that for many women this is the easiest position in which to be (multi-)orgasmic. Your partner can also keep the head of your penis in the most sensitive outer two inches of her vagina. It is difficult for a man to remain in only the first two inches when he is on top, since he tends to want to plunge deeper into the tighter area—which, of course, also finishes him off faster. In this position your partner can spiral her sacrum so that your penis rubs against the walls of her vagina at any depth and in any direction.

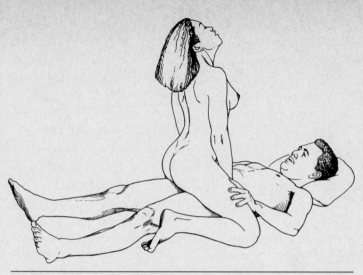

FIGURE 25. WOMAN-ON-TOP POSITION

In this position, you can also use your fingers to stimulate her clitoris and help her to climax. Another benefit of this position is that you can suck or fondle your partner's breasts while making love. According to the ancient Taoists, you can drink in your partner's sexual energy from her lips, her vagina, *and* her breasts.

This position is also especially good when the man is significantly larger than the woman or tends to ejaculate quickly, or when the woman is in the later months of pregnancy (her growing belly does not get squeezed). Older men and men with heart problems also find this position of great value, since they are not required to exert a lot of energy.

SIDE BY SIDE

This position requires relatively little exertion from either partner and is therefore good for later stages of lovemaking. It does require some skill to achieve and some coordination to maintain, so it is best for lovers who know each other well. It may be easiest to begin with you on top and for you to roll to the right or left into the side-by-side position. In addition to not requiring a great deal of strenuous effort, the position has the benefit of face-to-face and

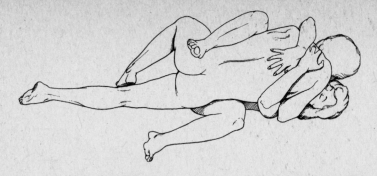

FIGURE 26. SIDE-BY-SIDE POSITION

whole-body contact, both of which allow for greater exchange of energy. However, it can be uncomfortable or awkward unless your partner's body movements and your own are well synchronized. And in this position the penetration of the penis is also quite shallow.

MAN FROM BEHIND

This is the way animals, whose main motivation is impregnation, do it, and with good reason. In this position, as you may have noticed, your partner's vagina feels especially tight, which makes ejaculatory control more difficult. This position is therefore best when you are feeling less aroused or have developed your skill at ejaculatory control. The reason your partner feels especially tight is that in this position you enter her deeply, which is the reason women who like especially deep penetration tend to favor this position. The depth can be controlled by your partner's angle: the more forward she bends, the deeper the penetration. This position is especially good for men with smaller penises or women with larger vaginas. This position also allows direct stimulation of your partner's G spot, although her clitoris receives relatively indirect stimulation—a situation you can remedy with your fingers.

Sexing the Spirit

It is no secret that most people experience transcendence more intensely in their bedrooms than they do in their churches, syna-

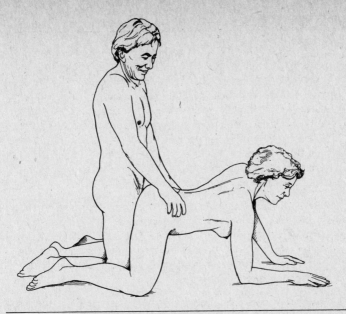

FIGURE 27. MAN-BEHIND POSITION

gogues, temples, or mosques. Lovemaking allows us to transcend the limits of our physical body, to fuse with another human being, and occasionally even to feel at one with the universe.

According to the Tao, heaven and earth are constantly in sexual union, balancing and harmonizing one another. When we make love we can connect with this universal energy. Healing Tao instructor Stefan Siegrist explained: "With Taoist sexuality one can reexperience the lost harmony (or spiritual oneness) with nature and the universe that is often talked about in philosophy and religion." Unlike some religions, however, Taoism views sexuality and spirituality as inseparable. Spirituality is "embodied," and spirit is seen as permeating the entire physical world, including our own bodies.

According to the Tao, each of us has three overlapping types of energy. In this book, we have been working primarily with the most physical of these three, our *ching-chi,* or sexual energy. But as we cultivate this sexual energy, it is refined into *chi,* or bioelectric energy (described in chapter 2), which then spreads throughout our entire body. And this in turn is refined into *shen,* or spiritual

SOUL-MATING (Exchanging Sexual Energy)

EXPANDING The pleasuring and thrusting and screwing techniques described earlier in this chapter will expand your and your partner's sexual energy to a point where it is ready to circulate. The more lubricated a woman is, the more yin energy she has. As we alluded to before, you can even drink her yin directly through oral sex or from the nipples of her breasts. It will help if you (and, ideally, your partner) have drawn the energy up and are circulating it through your own bodies (that is, through your Microcosmic Orbits).

EMBRACING Embrace your partner in a face-to-face position with most of your bodies in contact. If the woman is significantly lighter or weaker, she should be on top. Otherwise, it doesn't matter which person is on top. Remember to look deeply into each other's eyes: eye contact, as mentioned above, is extremely important. Send each other love and energy through your gaze.

BREATHING Coordinating your breathing is essential for exchanging *chi.* Now that you have stopped thrusting or screwing and are holding your partner close, place your nose next to your partner's ear and your ear next to your partner's nose. This will help you hear one another's breathing. Then synchronize your breathing: you can both inhale and exhale simultaneously, or one of you can inhale while the other exhales. Keep your thoughts focused on one another and be conscious of your chests rising and falling in rhythm with one another.

CIRCULATING To harmonize, both you and your partner must be able to circulate energy through your own Microcosmic Orbit as the first step toward balancing the Back Channel, which runs up your spine and is more yang, and the Front Channel, which runs down the front midline of your body and is more yin. Remember to draw energy up by contracting your anus and/or using your mind, and then to guide energy down the front of your body through your tongue.

EXCHANGING

1. After you have been breathing with one another for a while, you should each draw your energy from your genitals up to the crown of your head.

2. Then, while you are both inhaling, you should envision drawing her cool yin energy in from her vagina to your penis. (She should envision drawing your hot yang energy from your penis into her vagina.)

3. You should both continue drawing this energy back to your perineum and then up to your tailbone and finally up your spine to the crown of your head.

4. Then exhale and let the energy descend from the crown of your head through the midline between your eyebrows down your face and through your tongue—which, if your tongue is touching your partner's, will allow you to exchange energy through your mouths. From your tongue, the energy should be brought down the rest of your Front Channel to your navel. (You can also exchange energy from your heart through your chest to her breasts and from there down her Front Channel. She can do the same for you.)

5. Continue breathing and exchanging energy nine to eighteen times, or as long as you like.

energy. All three are interrelated and are connected to the body. In this section you will learn to circulate and refine your sexual energy with your partner. This technique will help you expand your orgasm from a purely physical experience to a spiritual one: this is the true nature of soul-mating.

YIN AND YANG

Most people who know anything about Taoism have heard about yin and yang and their complementary and cyclical positions in the symbol of the Tao. Most people know that yin is the *feminine* energy in the universe and that yang is its *masculine* counterpart. These two primordial energies are the electron and proton that allow all creation to occur and allow you and your partner to harmonize and refine your sexual energy. In the words of the *I Ching*, "The interaction of one yin and one yang is called Tao, and the resulting constant generative process is called 'change.'"[2]

According to Su Nü, "Yang can function only with the cooperation of

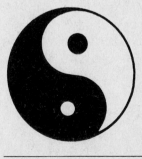

FIGURE 28. SYMBOL OF THE TAO

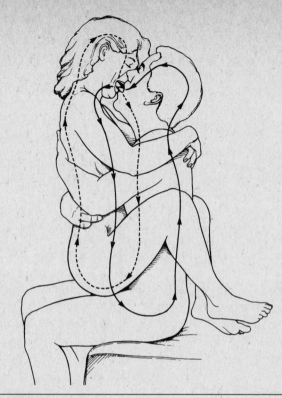

FIGURE 29. ENERGY EXCHANGE

yin, yin can grow only in the presence of yang." We have both masculine and feminine energies inside each of us, and yin and yang are dynamic forces that actually can change into one another. Many people
in the West now argue that *male* and *female* are simply socially con-
structed gender terms. According to the Tao, however, although there
is much variability from individual to individual, men generally have
more yang (masculine) energy and women generally have more yin
(feminine) energy. The Tao has always recognized that men are also
partly feminine and women also partly masculine and that any binary
opposition is clearly false. This idea is represented in the symbol of
the Tao by a small circle representing the masculine within the feminine symbol and a small circle representing the feminine within the
masculine symbol. Each contains a part of the other.

Though we should avoid binary opposition, we must be aware of our different needs, especially in the bedroom, or suffer the consequences. For example, yang is more quickly aroused and also more quickly extinguished; yin is more slowly aroused and more slowly extinguished. Because men tend to be more yang and women more yin, they also can help bring each other into better balance through the exchange of their energy during lovemaking. It is ideal if both partners are consciously aware of how this exchange takes place, and in the next chapter we explain what your partner will need to know about channeling her own energy. It is possible to feel the exchange of energy with a loving partner even if she does not know about Taoist sexuality, but it will be difficult to do exercise 13 without her active and informed participation. The more you can share with her, the easier and more powerful the exchange will be.

If you are having difficulty drawing your partner's energy up, you should contract your penis, your perineum, and your anus. Pumping these muscles lightly several times will help you draw the energy up. (You can also rhythmically sip up her energy with short breaths as in the Cool Draw exercise; see chapter 3.) Once you have good control over your sexual energy and are not worried about ejaculating, you can send your hot yang energy out your penis and into your partner. She in turn should imagine sending her cool yin energy from her vagina to your penis.

You cannot receive her yin energy without giving her your yang energy. Allowing her to absorb your excess yang energy will also help you avoid building up too much energy in your genitals and ejaculating. If you ejaculate, it is difficult to exchange energy, because you lose most of yours. Remember, it is the exchange that is important.

You will probably not be able to open all the points along the spine during your first exchange of sexual energy. It may take many times—it may even take months—but eventually you will feel the warm current between your mouths and between your genitals. "Sometimes," described one multi-orgasmic man, "when we are both orgasming we will be kissing passionately and will feel the energy going right through the both of us. Just driving through our tongues, down my body, through my penis, into her vagina, and up through her body back to our tongues. It is incredible."

At first the energy may seem so explosive that you have a hard time distinguishing between your and your partner's energy. However, eventually you will be able to distinguish between your partner's cool yin energy and your hot yang energy. If your partner does not know how to circulate her own energy, you can help her by guiding the energy from your penis to her vagina, up her spine to her crown, down to her tongue and yours, and then back down her front to her vagina.

FINDING THE WAY

Spontaneous Energy Movements

Don't be surprised if at first the energy moves spontaneously and unpredictably. You may experience energy rising up the front midline of your bodies between you and your partner. Some couples experience energy shooting to the top of their heads and showering down over them, while others report feeling surrounded by a cocoon of energy. If you experience any of these, don't get worried. Just relax and enjoy the movement of these subtle energies through or around your bodies.

CULTIVATING YOUR ENERGY

After considerable practice, you will be able to open ever higher centers of energy, called *tan-tien* (or reservoirs; pronounced *DON TYEN*) by the Chinese. According to Taoism, one of these reservoirs exists at the level of your navel, another at your heart, and a third at your head (see figure 3). Michael Winn explains: "While in actual fact the entire body is one large interconnected *tan tien*, or field of energy, it is easiest to try to open each center sequentially. You must open the lower centers first to provide a strong platform for the higher ones."

Some yoga-trained Westerners confuse these reservoirs with the Hindu chakras, which have become popular synonyms for energy centers in the body. The seven or twelve chakras are generally more local and separated than the *tan-tien,* which are part of one large energy circuit, the Microcosmic Orbit, that envelops the entire body. Although Hindu Tantric philosophy is similar in many ways to Taoism, especially in its emphasis on conserving and transforming the power of sperm, the specific methods used in Tantra are different.

BECOMING ONE

This mutual opening of the Microcosmic Orbits of two lovers is the true fusion of sexual and spiritual energy. It can eventually result, after refining your sexual energy through elevated lovemaking and through meditation, in a prolonged orgasm and even an altered state of consciousness. According to Taoism, this orgasmic fusion of lovers occurs when yin and yang are in complete harmony. The more you learn to relax and to surrender yourself completely to your partner, the more likely it is that you will experience this extraordinary connection. According to one multi-orgasmic man, "Sex with my girlfriend is not the mechanical battle of bodies groping for momentary pleasure that it was, but a real exchange and a real union of our two bodies—almost as if our two bodies were merging into one."

This form of harmonizing is very powerful. When you can open and receive the loving energy of your partner, and in turn have your partner open to receive your energy, you will experience a blending and intimacy unlike anything else. Both of your energies, yin and yang, are part of the same universal energy; they are just charged differently. This is how you and your partner can truly become one flesh. When this flow of sexual energy between you reaches the right intensity and balance, your individual bodies will seem to dissolve into the ecstatic vibration of your circulating and pulsating energies. This is a true orgasm of body and soul. Assuming that other channels of communication and sharing are open in your relationship, this exchange of energy will help your love grow, and your mutual love will enrich those around you.

We often call healthy sexual union *making love*, and this is exactly what you are doing. Sexual energy expands and intensifies our emotions and attitudes. This is why sexual pleasure is popularly considered the highest bliss, and why the feeling of being in love is so intense and all-encompassing. On the negative side, it is also why lovers' quarrels are the most intense. So it is of paramount importance that you and your partner try to resolve emotional conflicts *before* you attempt to circulate sexual energy. Put another way, sexual energy is like fire: it can cook your food, and it can also burn your house down. It all depends on how it is used. If negative emotions arise while you are making love, stop or try to transform them into positive emotions by smiling and thinking about the positive qualities of your partner.

A genuine smile transmits loving energy, which has the power to warm and to heal. Recall a time when you were upset or physically ill and someone gave you a big smile; suddenly you felt better. Norman Cousins, a former editor of the *Saturday Review*, writes in *Anatomy of an Illness* that he cured himself of a rare connective-tissue disease by watching old Marx Brothers movies. Smiling and laughter have the ability to transform negative energy into positive energy and to heal our bodies and minds. If you have a lot of negativity in general, you should try practicing the Inner Smile and the Six Healing Sounds, which are described in Mantak Chia's book *Taoist Ways to Transform Stress into Vitality* (see the appendix).

When to Stop

As we mentioned in chapter 3, most couples stop making love when the man ejaculates. There may be some cuddling or, during new hot and steamy relationships, another round of lovemaking after a refractory period (the time it takes to get another erection once you have ejaculated). But most people call it a night (or a morning or an afternoon) once the man ejaculates. As you may have guessed, with non-ejaculatory, multi-orgasmic sex, this ordinary end marker no longer exists. You and your partner can make love as long as you want.

Though, as we mentioned earlier, Taoist sexuality should not be an endurance test, when time allows, you may wish to spend an hour or two or more in a passionate and harmonizing embrace. (*Don't forget to let your erection decrease some around every twenty minutes so the blood can recirculate.*) The classic Taoist texts suggest that it takes one thousand loving thrusts to fully satisfy a woman. This may seem to involve an awful lot of effort and to demand great physical strength, but as Jolan Chang points out in his *Tao of Love and Sex,* if half an hour's run requires at least two thousand steps, why shouldn't prolonged lovemaking involve a thousand or more thrusts? Of course, for most of us, our lives do not afford the time for this kind of intense session every night, and no couple will want such intensity all the time. However, to reach the higher levels of orgasmic and energizing lovemaking, it is important to set aside times when the phone is off the hook so that you and you partner can discover your true potential for pleasure. It's certainly better than going to the movies!

If your partner generally has more desire than you, Sexual Kung Fu may help save your love life. It will increase your sexual energy significantly and allow you to satisfy your partner's desire with ease. Though for most women one thousand loving thrusts will be paradise, for others with less sexual desire it may be purgatory. If your partner generally has less desire than you, she should definitely read the next chapter and try to expand her passion and her pleasure. Of course, if there are deeper psychological reasons that prevent either of you from expressing your sexual selves fully, you should seek help from a professional therapist. The ability of both partners to have multiple orgasms is a powerful aphrodisiac, but real, lasting satisfaction comes from a relationship based on sexual and emotional harmony.

How you end lovemaking is as important as how you start. As we explained in chapter 1, the loss of energy that most men experience after ejaculating makes it difficult for them to remain attentive and affectionate toward their partners. Since female sexuality is less precipitous, most women want to disengage more gradually, with tender words and caresses. As you master Sexual Kung Fu, you will no longer fall off the ejaculatory cliff and will be able to conclude lovemaking more gradually.

One multi-orgasmic man explained his experience: "Before, I didn't understand or want the kind of caressing and love talk after sex that my girlfriend did. Once I had had my ejaculation, I had no desire to caress my partner, to talk to her, or even to kiss her. But now during and even *after* lovemaking I have a deep desire to caress her body and to be tender to her. Her skin often feels like it is tingling with an electrical charge, which makes it soft like silk."

If your partner is (or becomes) multi-orgasmic, you will find that you can ride the waves of orgasm together for as long as you like, tuning your passion and your pleasure. If your partner is not multi-orgasmic, or even orgasmic, one thousand loving thrusts will give her the best possible chance of becoming so. More important, Taoist sexuality allows you to experience a profound intimacy that is difficult to describe in words and impossible to count in orgasms.

When to Start: A Few Words About Safer Sex

In his stand-up routine about sexually transmitted diseases, comedian Eddie Murphy echoed the general cultural anxiety around sex today: "AIDS, that ain't like the good old days when venereal disease was simple. In the good old days ya got gonorrhea, your dick hurt, you go get a shot—clear it right up. Then they came out with herpes. You keep that shit forever—like luggage. Now they got AIDS, that just kills motherfuckers. I say, What's next? I guess you just put your dick in and it explodes."

It is difficult to focus on the greater pleasure, intimacy, and spiritual growth possible through sexuality when you are worried about the health of your and your partner's physical body. For this reason, it is worth discussing the realities and logistics of safer sex. You may also be relieved to know that according to the Tao, when you practice Sexual Kung Fu and don't ejaculate, you greatly strengthen your immune system. You also obviously reduce the risk of exchanging a sexually transmitted disease through bodily fluids.

AIDS—acquired immune deficiency syndrome—is the disease that results from infection by the human immunodeficiency virus (HIV). Although AIDS is not the only sexually transmitted disease you need to be concerned about, it is certainly the most dangerous. AIDS is currently thought to be universally fatal, although it is not clear whether all people who are living with HIV will eventually develop AIDS. Those who die from AIDS usually do so because their immune system is so compromised that they cannot fight the opportunistic infections that often accompany AIDS.

HIV is spread through bodily fluids—specifically, blood and semen. There is no evidence so far to suggest that HIV can be transmitted through saliva. Sexual practices that are safe or very low risk include hugging, massage, dry kissing (without exchanging saliva), and mutual masturbation. Sexual practices that are probably safe include French kissing, fellatio (without ejaculation), cunnilingus, and vaginal and anal intercourse with a condom.

Though the two main groups at risk are homosexual or bisexual men and intravenous drug users, heterosexual men and women are also at risk.[3] This fact has created an atmosphere of panic that, although valuable in mobilizing the medical community and helping raise awareness about the importance of sexual education, has left most people with bedroom jitters.

Asking potential partners whether they have had an AIDS test or inquiring about their sexual history is as much a part of dating these days as asking about their employment or relatives. Many couples are getting tested for AIDS together. Although not yet considered a romantic date, getting tested is one way for couples to express their love and concern for one another's health and well-being.

Safer sex is recommended for any couple in which one partner could have been exposed to HIV. Couples interested in getting sexually involved should first have an HIV test, then use safer-sex techniques for six months, and then get a confirming HIV test. (It may take up to six months after infection for a person to test positive.) If both tests are negative, chances are very, very low that there is any more reason for concern, so long as the couple remains monogamous.

In the six months during which couples are waiting to take a second HIV test, they can engage in safer-sex techniques such as intercourse with a condom and mutual masturbation. In addition, they can each practice solo-cultivation techniques to develop their individual sexual and spiritual potential. Not only can using your hands to satisfy one another, a technique we mentioned earlier, allow you to have safer sex during the six-month waiting period, but it can also allow each of you to learn the subtle nuances of your individual arousal and pleasure that will help you become multi-orgasmic. Interrupting the routine also can allow you to explore new sensual and sexual pleasures while avoiding old coital scripts. Most important, harmonizing with your partner, according to the Tao, occurs at an energetic level that does not require intercourse. Caressing and even mutual meditation when gazing into one another's eyes can be profoundly intimate and satisfying experiences.

SAFER SAFER SEX

By not ejaculating, the man does not transfer as much bodily fluid (and, potentially, as many bacteria and viruses) to the woman. Also, by not ejaculating he does not draw in as much fluid (and, potentially, as many bacteria and viruses) from the woman. If you can excuse the comparison, your penis is a little like a turkey baster. When you ejaculate, you squeeze out your semen, creating a low-pressure vacuum, which then draws in liquid from your partner. By not creating this vacuum, you have less chance of transferring bacteria or viruses to or from your partner.

During nonejaculatory sex, bodily fluids can still be transferred (which is also the reason nonejaculatory sex alone is not a reliable birth-control technique). Still, nonejaculatory sex is safer than ejaculatory sex, especially if the condom breaks. (It also makes whatever birth-control method you use all the more effective.)

FINDING THE WAY

The Art and Science of Using Condoms

The good news about condoms is that the decreased sensitivity that most men experience can help a man control his ejaculation. The bad news about condoms is that they *do* decrease a man's sensitivity. Some men actually have difficulty keeping an erection while wearing a condom. If this is your situation, you or your partner should keep stroking your genitals while you put on the condom. Putting a small amount of lubricant on your penis before putting on the condom will also increase your sensitivity without causing the condom to slip off. Following are a few other things to keep in mind when using condoms.

1. Always use a condom before vaginal or anal intercourse. Also, try to use a condom with spermicide that contains nonoxynol-9, which is effective in killing a variety of sexually transmitted diseases, including HIV. (If you develop a bright red inflammation on your penis or vulva as a reaction to nonoxynol-9, switch to a brand without this germicide, but be extra careful.)

2. Always use a condom before your partner performs oral sex. In this case, your partner will probably want you to use a "dry" condom that is not lubricated and does not have nonoxynol-9, which has a medicinal taste.

3. Leave half an inch of space at the top of plain-tip condoms. Reservoir-tip condoms are designed to create this space. Make sure that the condom covers your entire penis, and smooth the condom to squeeze out any air bubbles. If you are uncircumcised, pull back your foreskin before putting on the condom. If the condom starts to slip off, you can hold it on with your fingers.

4. Apply plenty of lubricant to the outside of the condom. (Not putting on enough lubricant is one of the major reasons that condoms break.) Use only *water-based* lubricants such as K-Y jelly or Astroglide.

Petroleum-based lubricants such as Vaseline can cause latex condoms, dams, or gloves to disintegrate.

5. After intercourse, withdraw while you are still erect and hold the base of the condom to make sure it does not slip off. Throw away the condom and, especially if you have ejaculated, wash off your penis or put on a new condom before continuing to caress one another.

6. A condom generally slips off or breaks because it wasn't put on correctly, because sex was "too" vigorous, or because the condom was not held during withdrawal. If the condom breaks or comes off and you have not ejaculated or if the tear is near the base of the condom, you probably don't need to worry. Just remove the broken condom and put on a new one. If the condom breaks and you have ejaculated, safer-sex experts recommend that your partner urinate and insert spermicidal foam or jelly into her vagina to help destroy the sperm, viruses, and bacteria. She should leave the spermicide there for at least an hour. If you and your partner are concerned that she will get pregnant, your partner may wish to take the "morning after" pill, which she can obtain from her physician.

THE POWER TO CREATE AND DESTROY

The ease with which AIDS and other sexually transmitted diseases spread is the pathological reminder of an essential Taoist insight into the nature of sexual intimacy: lovemaking is a physical and energetic exchange that can profoundly influence the health and well-being of both partners. In our Western emphasis on individuality and independence we have forgotten about this interdependence and interpenetration. The sexual revolution did not fully take into account the significance of this exchange. As sexually transmitted diseases such as herpes and AIDS will not let us forget, we are deeply affected by our sexual histories.

Although Western medicine recognizes that bacteria and viruses can be transmitted during intercourse, it has yet to recognize the rest of the biochemical and energetic exchange that takes place during sex. According to the Taoists, every time you and your partner make love you exchange hormones, enzymes, vitamins, and so on through your sexual secretions. This seems straightforward enough. Through the entwining of your bodies and your engorged genitals, the Taoists also believe, you exchange much more—physically, emotionally, and spiritually. It may be some time before Western science can distill and quantify the various components of this exchange, but if you practice Sexual Kung Fu, you will have the proof of this exchange in your own body.

Caution is an important response to the AIDS epidemic, but the fear that stalks our bedrooms misses the point. Sexuality has always been powerful; intercourse has always had the potential for miraculous creation or tragic destruction. Sex can heal us or hurt us. Respect and even awe, rather than fear, are the appropriate components of a healthy attitude toward sexuality, which the Taoists have always known was the true alchemy, the source of our life and health.

Satisfaction Guaranteed

For Women

This chapter is written for you as the female partner of a man who is practicing Sexual Kung Fu. (*Kung fu* literally means "practice," so *Sexual Kung Fu* simply means "sexual practice.") This chapter will give you a brief explanation of what Taoist sexuality is and how it can help you and your partner have a more pleasurable, healthier, and more intimate love life. Although this is meant to be a self-contained chapter that you can read without consulting the rest of the book, you may find it helpful to read as many of the other chapters as you can, especially chapters 4, 5, and 9, which are for couples. (Though there is some repetition here from other chapters, men who are reading this book may also want to read this chapter as a way to review what they have already learned and to discover what is most important for their partner to know.)

Multiple Orgasms for Men?

The fact that men can have multiple orgasms is still so shocking to most of us, women and men alike, that you may find it hard to believe. As we mentioned in the introduction, it is worth remembering that only in the last forty years have female multiple orgasms been recognized and accepted as normal. Even more incredible is the number of women who have become multi-orgasmic—once they realized it was possible. Since the fifties, when Alfred Kinsey was conducting his famous studies of human sexuality, the percentage of women who experience multiple orgasms has tripled, from 14 percent to over 50 percent.[1]

In the 1980s, sexologists William Hartman and Marilyn Fithian found that about 12 percent of the men they studied were multi-orgasmic. As your partner begins to recognize that he also has this potential and as you help him learn some simple techniques, he too will experience multiple orgasms. One partner of a multi-orgasmic man recalled: "The first time my boyfriend had an orgasm without ejaculating I couldn't believe it. He was clearly experiencing as much pleasure as usual and I could feel his penis pulsating, but much to my surprise there was no semen and moments later we were able to continue making love. It's still amazing to me that he can have such intense orgasms without ejaculating. Now I am surprised when he does ejaculate." Another partner of a multi-orgasmic man described what she experiences when her partner has an orgasm without ejaculating: "My partner stops moving for a moment and moans and trembles. I can feel the strong throbbing of his penis deep inside me. Ordinarily that would be it, but not now."

Yet multiple orgasms are just the beginning. In the West, we tend to see the "big O" as the be-all and end-all of sexuality, and many women spend a great deal of time worrying about whether they are orgasmic, when they are orgasmic, and how they are orgasmic. In Taoist sexuality, experiencing an orgasm, one or many, is not the goal. These peaks of pleasure are just part of an ecstatic process of lovemaking. Once you and your partner learn to circulate sexual energy through your bodies, you can experience orgasmic waves of pleasure as often as you like. When you make love, you will experience a depth of intimacy—a physical, emotional, and even spiritual bond—that you may have rarely, if ever, felt before.

Why Me? Why Him? Why This?

Any kind of self-improvement, sexual as much as any other, requires some effort, and this book is written to teach your partner and you in clear, simple terms how to deepen your sexual lives and your relationship to one another.

If your partner has given you this chapter (or book) to read, you may be somewhat skeptical about this newfangled sexual practice and wonder why you (and he) need it. You should know that the Tao (pronounced *DOW*) of sexuality is anything but new. It is at least a three-thousand-year-old tradition of accumulated wisdom recording how people can make love most pleasurably and most healthfully. Even the most seasoned lover can probably learn something from this treasure trove of experience. Interestingly, in the Taoist tradition most of the sex advisers (including the emperor's own consultants) were women. How different from the West, where until recently almost all sex advice was given by men—if given at all.

Especially if your sexual relationship is already rich and satisfying, you may be wondering why you need to read a book about "doing what comes naturally." Though all people have instinctual sexual desire, what we do with this desire and how we maintain and cultivate it over a lifetime are anything but obvious. In the West, we take for granted that couples will lose their passion for one another over the years, but according to the Tao this is not a law of nature and in fact this attraction never needs to wither. (We talk more about this in the final chapter, "Making Love for a Lifetime.")

If you bought this book for your partner or to learn more about male sexuality, you may be very eager to help your lover become multi-orgasmic. Nonetheless, you may feel that you spend too much time trying to please your partner, and certainly there are many women who do just that. This book, however, is not about your pleasing him. One of the main benefits of Taoist sexuality is that it teaches your partner how he can cultivate his sexual skill and how he can better please you. Though this book is entitled *The*

Multi-Orgasmic Man, it could just as well have been called *The Multi-Orgasmic Couple.* In the words of one partner of a multi-orgasmic man, "When my husband started practicing Sexual Kung Fu, I began experiencing multiple orgasms much more often. This is a *very* special gift."

LASTING PLEASURE

In our society, women are told that they need to please their men sexually. In Taoist sexuality, a great many of the techniques were developed to help men please women. In the end, however, one partner's pleasure is inseparable from the other's, according to the Tao. The stereotype of marital relations in our society is of the frigid wife and the ever-desirous husband, but the truth is that there are many women who are more interested in making love than their partners, especially if their partners are being exhausted by sex that focuses on ejaculation.

As we discussed in chapter 1, the image of the unsatisfied woman whose lover ejaculates, grunts, and collapses on top of her is so common it has become a cultural joke. It is no wonder that many women lose interest in sex that is frenetic and lacks real connection, physical and emotional. This, too, is a stereotype, and all surveys show that in recent years men have been trying harder to please their partners and to last longer in bed.[2]

Your lover probably does not grunt or collapse on top of you if he is interested enough in his and your sexuality to read this book, but Taoist masters have long known that it is difficult for men to maintain an interest in satisfying their partners or in being intimate once they have ejaculated. One multi-orgasmic man explained his experience: "After I ejaculated I didn't want to and didn't understand her need to caress and talk after sex. Now that I don't ejaculate, after lovemaking I love for us to lie together and caress each other slowly, almost in sort of a meditation."

BEYOND THE BIG BANG

Fortunately, the Taoists also discovered almost three thousand years ago that orgasm and ejaculation are not the same thing and that men can have orgasms (in fact, multiple orgasms) without ejaculating. This is possible because orgasm and ejaculation are two distinct physical processes, as has more recently been confirmed by Western medical science (see chapters 1 and 2). The partner of a multi-orgasmic man explained how her husband changed once he learned to orgasm without ejaculating: "My husband used to get tired quickly after he ejaculated. And sometimes he would want to drink alcohol and he would tend to get impatient or annoyed easily. Now he is so energetic and loving."

Male sexuality in the West remains incorrectly focused on the inevitably disappointing goal of ejaculation ("getting off") instead of on the orgasmic process of lovemaking. *The Multi-Orgasmic Man* teaches your partner how to separate orgasm and ejaculation in his own body, allowing him to move beyond focusing on the momentary release of ejaculation and to cultivate longer-lasting and more profound levels of sexual pleasure with you. Taoist sexuality will allow your partner to be more sensitive to your body as he becomes more sensitive to his own. By moving beyond the Big Bang theory of sexuality, which has often left women unsatisfied, it also allows men and women to harmonize their sexuality for ever-higher levels of intimacy and ecstasy.

SEXUAL HEALING

Sexual pleasure is, however, just one part of feeling good. Taoist sexuality can also help you and your partner stay healthier and possibly even, believe it or not, live longer. Sexual Kung Fu began as a branch of Chinese medicine, and the ancient Taoists were themselves doctors. As physicians they were concerned as much with the body's physical well-being as they were with its sexual satisfaction. Sexuality was seen as the most potent medicine, both curative and preventive. If you were sick, a Taoist doctor might very well prescribe—in addition to herbs and acupuncture—a two-week regimen of lovemaking in certain positions. Now that's (to quote Aretha Franklin) Dr. Feel Good in the Morning.

There are other, more obvious benefits. With nonejaculatory lovemaking—in which the man orgasms but does not ejaculate—whatever birth control you use will be even more effective. Equally as important in these days of sexually transmitted diseases and concern over the transfer of bodily fluids, nonejaculatory sex is also safer sex. Whatever other safer-sex precautions you take (using a condom, to take an obvious example) will be all the safer if your partner is not ejaculating.

An added benefit is that nonejaculatory sex is less messy—no more wet spots or arguing over who has to sleep on them. Many women also appreciate not having their partner's semen dripping out of their vagina. As one partner of a multi-orgasmic man put it, "My vagina felt like it was sparkling with my own secretions. I liked not having his sperm dripping out of me all night."

The kind of profound sexual intimacy that Taoist sexuality allows is not a relationship cure-all, or a replacement for other forms of communication, but it can deepen your love. Open and honest communication is an essential part of this practice, and it won't work if you just grin and bear it. There will be moments, as your partner is learning to control his ejaculation, when he asks you to stop moving or to help in some other way, but in general this momentary sacrifice will be rewarded with many, many more moments, minutes, hours of pleasure. However, sex should never be a sacrifice one partner makes for the other, and if necessary, he can always practice the techniques in this book on his own. This "solo cultivation" is an important part of the practice and is not regarded with the same stigma that is associated with masturbation in the West. The most important factor in your partner's ability to become multi-orgasmic and in your and his ability to become a multi-orgasmic couple is your support and your sincere desire.

Helping Your Partner Become Multi-Orgasmic

The first thing you need to do before you can help your partner is overcome any resistance you may have to wanting him to become multi-orgasmic or to his doing the Sexual Kung Fu practice.

WILL OUR LOVEMAKING BECOME MECHANICAL?   At first many women worry that lovemaking with their partner will become mechanical. As Dr. Barbara Keesling points out in her recent book, *How to Make Love All Night (And Drive a Woman Wild)*, many women fear that the techniques for becoming multi-orgasmic that their partners learn will "turn their stud into a mechanical bull." She testifies that the experience takes a man "into his body, not away from it." As a sex therapist and former sex surrogate who has trained over one hundred men to become multi-orgasmic, she speaks from personal as well as professional experience.

Like learning to play a musical instrument, learning Sexual Kung Fu will take some time and effort and may be a little awkward at first. The best approach is to relax and have fun with it. One multi-orgasmic man described how Taoist sexuality can relax the tension that often exists around sexuality: "It is fun to talk about it; it is fun to laugh about it. It can relax the whole bedroom tension. Because I am talking frankly about my body, women will talk about theirs. I was with one woman who I was telling about my practice and all of a sudden she pulled out her vibrator, and she said, 'I was never going to show this to anyone because I've been so uptight about my sexuality. But I feel I can share anything with you because you were able to share this with me.' And that was really cool."

Most men learn about sex through masturbation and pornography. For whatever reasons—guilt, inexperience, fear of getting caught—most men learn to masturbate quickly. Pornography also generally takes men away from their bodies. It is no surprise then that most men are not very connected to their bodies or aware of their arousal rates. Taoist sexuality teaches men to learn their body's true potential to experience pleasure and to pleasure their partners. Although at first your partner will need to concentrate on learning to control his arousal rate and his urge to ejaculate, once he has this control he will be much better able to concentrate on you and on the profound process of lovemaking you are both engaged in.

DOESN'T A MAN NEED TO EJACULATE TO BE TRULY SATISFIED?
Some women feel that pleasing their man means helping him ejaculate. This feeling is not surprising since most men do ejaculate at the end of lovemaking and many women hear from their first partners during the fever of adolescent petting that they will have pain in their genitals (often called *blue balls* or *lover's nuts*) if they don't ejaculate. This may be true for the bumping and grinding that

often occurs during adolescence, but when your partner practices Sexual Kung Fu, he will no longer have the same need to ejaculate. One multi-orgasmic man explained: "Sometimes during lovemaking, especially if it was long and beautiful, my girlfriend wanted me to ejaculate. Still, I usually didn't ejaculate, and later she would see that there was no need for me to ejaculate and that I could much more deeply satisfy her and myself if I didn't."

After years of having lovemaking concluded by your partner's ejaculating, however, you may have feelings about his no longer ejaculating every time. At first some women feel that they are less sexy or less capable lovers. Although this feeling is understandable, it is certainly not the case that they are any less sexy or capable, and it won't take long for you to see that your real success as a lover is dependent not on your partner's ejaculation but on his— and your—pleasure.

GETTING HIM HOT

Before you begin learning specific techniques to help your partner, there are a few basics you should know about male sexuality, if you don't already. This section is meant as a brief overview. A longer discussion of the subject appears in chapter 2. (Also, you will find figure 2 on page 12 useful in figuring out where everything is.) We tend to think of male sexuality as the penis—and what could be complex or hidden about this most obvious of organs? But the penis is really just the beginning.

Although most men can learn to experience sensation throughout their entire bodies through the whole-body orgasms described in this book, most of a man's sexual sensitivity remains, at least initially, in his groin. As Dr. Alex Comfort writes in his *The New Joy of Sex,* "Genital approach is how men get into the mood." Lampoon it, rail against it, or excuse it, but the truth is, that's the way it is for most men. The genitals are of central importance to most male sexuality, but the genitals are not simply the penis.

Besides the penis itself, and especially the head of the penis, which has the most nerve endings, the testicles are often very sensitive for a man (although they must be treated more gently than the penis). It is important to keep in mind that your partner may not get an erection or may even lose his erection when his testicles are being stimulated. This does not mean he is not experiencing intense pleasure, but the lack or loss of an erection can often cause him or you to worry. Your conveying to him that you know this is a normal part of his arousal will help him lay these fears to rest.

It is worth keeping in mind that when a man lies on his back, gravity draws blood away from his erection. If your partner is having trouble getting or maintaining an erection, it is best for him *not* to be on his back. You can also help him get an erection by encircling the base of his penis with your thumb and forefinger. By squeezing these together in a snug ring, you can help prevent the blood from leaving his erection as you stimulate him with your other hand or mouth.

The perineum, the area between the testicles and anus, is also highly sensitive. The anus, too, is very sensitive, but for many men—as for many women—it is taboo, so approach slowly or ask first. The inner thighs can also be very responsive. Many men also enjoy nipple stimulation and experience nipple erections just like women. Some require persistent, regular stimulation to awaken these nerves, while others never warm to this touch no matter how much they (or you) try.

It is also worth remembering that a man's erection is directly connected to his self-esteem. The famous fragile male ego is all the more fragile in bed. Most men know very little about the bedroom arts and not only worry about what they don't know but feel they are supposed to know everything. As a result, it is best to try not to criticize. If your partner is doing something you don't like, tell him what you would like him to do rather than criticize what he is doing wrong. (Later, away from the heat of passion, you can for future reference tell him what you don't like. Developing an open channel of communication about sex away from the bedroom is very important for a healthy sex life.) Finally, the sound of a woman's genuine pleasure is the greatest aphrodisiac. The more you can share your enjoyment with him, the more he'll know what you like and the more excited he will become. Your sexual pleasure will expand his, as his will yours.

COOLING HIM OFF

Now that we've discussed how to get your partner all hot and bothered, it's time to learn how to cool him off. This is the real challenge for most men, and anything you can do to help will be much appreciated. You can tell when he is approaching the point of no return ("ejaculatory inevitability") by reading his bodily signs. Before your partner can ejaculate, his scrotum will have to draw in close to his body. (This happens less as men get older.) The muscles in his thighs and stomach may also become tense and his body rigid, and his voice or breathing may change.

STOPPING The most important thing you can do to help him keep from going beyond the point of no return is to stop moving when he signals with his voice or body that he is getting too close. Male orgasm takes place just before the precipice of ejaculation. For your partner to become multi-orgasmic, he must learn to experience an orgasm without falling over the edge of ejaculation.

Imagine that your partner is in a hang glider. He is running toward a cliff, and he must learn to take off and soar into nonejaculatory orgasms just before he falls down the steep slope of ejaculation. If you move when he is close to the edge, you may push him over and down into the ravine of postejaculatory stupor. If you are able to stop for a moment while he regains control of his arousal, you will be able to soar together. If he goes over the cliff, he will be lying on the rocks below just as you are ready to take off.

ASKING Helping your partner to be aware of his arousal and his proximity to the point of no return will also help him at first. This does not mean you have to be detached or act as an observer, but simply that you let him know if you notice he is getting too close to the edge. One multi-orgasmic man described how his partner helps: "My girlfriend will ask whether I am close if she sees that I am. And that really helps remind me to be aware of my arousal. You might think that talking about how close I am would interrupt lovemaking, but it never does. It makes it fuller because there is more sharing, there is better communication, which is the key to any relationship whether you are in the bedroom or not."

ENCOURAGING   It is better to focus on the process of love-making than on not ejaculating. As one multi-orgasmic man explained, "My wife would say, 'Don't come yet.' Well, that would make me ejaculate more quickly because I would be focusing on ejaculating. What we found is that when she says, 'I feel good' or 'This is great!' this stroking, if you will, of the male ego helps me regain my control and not ejaculate." Any successful coach tells her team what they should do, not what they shouldn't, since the body is more likely to do what the mind is thinking about.

BREATHING   Your partner will also be using his breathing to help him control his arousal. When he gets close to ejaculating, he may breathe deeply and slowly or shallowly and quickly. The first helps him control his sexual energy and the second helps him disperse it. Whichever he finds works for him, it is very helpful if you remind him to breathe or breathe with him. Harmonizing your and his breathing is also part of the couples practice we discuss in chapter 5, which can help the two of you connect with one another more deeply.

CIRCULATING   The most important technique your partner will be using to delay ejaculation is the pumping of his sexual energy away from his genitals and up through his spine to the rest of his body. If the sexual energy continues to build up in his groin, it will eventually be too great to control and will shoot out in the most direct way it can—through his penis. However, if he draws this energy away, it will be much easier for him to stop his urge to ejaculate.

Learning to circulate energy through the body is the secret to whole-body orgasms for both of you. You can help your partner circulate his sexual energy by running your hands up his spine from his tailbone to his head, helping him to draw the energy up. In general, as Senior Healing Tao instructor Michael Winn explains, "The more a woman can touch and stroke a man's whole body and help him be less penis oriented, the easier it will be for him to move the energy out of his penis and to other parts of his body." Circulating energy yourself can help intensify your own orgasms and energize you. It will also help you to experience greater intimacy and ecstasy together.

The techniques we have described are essential for helping your partner keep his cool when you are in the throes of passionate lovemaking. You or your partner can also use a number of more mechanical techniques to help him avoid ejaculating as well.

SQUEEZING The *squeeze* technique was originally developed for men who ejaculate "prematurely." (If your partner ejaculates quickly, be sure you and he read the section called "It's Not Over Till It's Over: Ending Premature Ejaculation" in chapter 8.) The squeeze technique is quite simple: when your partner is getting close to ejaculating, you can place your thumb on the underside of his penis and squeeze. Another method is for one of you to grip his penis as you would the handlebar of a bicycle and to press your thumb down on the tip (see figure 8b on page 50). You or he can also squeeze the base of his penis between your thumb and first two fingers. Any of these methods will help your partner stop the urge to ejaculate and draw his sexual energy out of his penis and away from his genitals.

The obvious problem with the squeeze technique is that you need to stop intercourse and your partner will need to pull out. In the past, women who practiced the Tao were able to use their vaginal (what we now call the PC) muscle to squeeze the head of their partner's penis, which would also help prevent him from ejaculating. You may want to experiment with this technique as well after reading the section later in this chapter called "Strengthening Your Sex Muscle."

PRESSING The Taoist sages discovered a spot on the perineum, called the Million-Dollar Point, that they found was extremely helpful in stopping men from ejaculating. It was originally called the Million-Gold-Piece Point because that is what it cost a man to have a Taoist master show him where it was. (The Taoist sages were not too holy to get paid.) Your partner's Million-Dollar Point is located just in front of his anus (see figure 2 on page 12). There should be an indentation at the correct spot. If your partner presses his finger into this spot and contracts his PC muscle, he can help delay ejaculation by focusing his attention and interrupting his ejaculatory reflex. It is important for you to know what he is doing if he starts pushing on his perineum during lovemaking. If you and your partner know each other's bodies well and have a lot of experience in bed together, you can help him delay ejaculation by pressing on this spot during intercourse. You will need to push your finger in up to about your first joint. It is necessary to apply firm (although not too hard), consistent pressure for a moment or two.

Once he has passed the point of no return, your partner can also press on this spot while squeezing his PC muscle to stop the semen from leaving his body and thus avoid losing all of the hormones and nutrients in his semen (we discuss the reasons for his wanting to avoid losing semen in chapter 1). This more complex manipulation, which we call the Finger Lock and describe in chapter 3, is probably best left up to him, but you should know what he is up to. If he uses the Finger Lock to conserve his semen, he will still lose his erection, but many men report that it returns more quickly. Keep in mind that the Finger Lock should not be used as a form of birth control or safer sex, since some semen may leak out.

You can also press your finger rhythmically at the Million-Dollar Point, an action that mimics the prostate contractions he experiences during orgasm and that can be very pleasurable for your partner. However, this rhythmic pressure should *not* be used when he is close to the edge, for it will very likely push him over into ejaculation.

PULLING   Because your partner's testicles have to pull up close to his body in order for the semen to be propelled out of the testes, pulling them away from the body can delay his ejaculating. You can help him by gently pulling down on his testicles. Circle your thumb and forefinger just as you did earlier to help him maintain his erection. Instead of circling the base of his penis, however, this time you will circle the top of his testicles (see figure 9 on page 51). Then you will pull down firmly. (Remember, a man's testicles are extremely sensitive and should be handled with care.)

The more you support your partner's practice, the easier it will be for him and the better your lovemaking will become. As a woman, your sexual ability is naturally stronger than your partner's. The Taoists compare a man's sexual arousal to fire and a woman's to water. Fire is easily ignited but easily extinguished. Water is slow to boil but able to maintain its heat for a long time. Water is always stronger than fire and can easily quench it. The Taoists strive to teach men how they can last long enough to bring their partner's desire to the boiling point. This ability, they know, is the basis for sexual satisfaction for both partners. In addition to helping your partner control his fire, you can also learn to help bring yourself to the boiling point. Whether you are currently preorgasmic, orgasmic, or multi-orgasmic, the most important thing you can do to help your partner and yourself is to cultivate your own sexuality and to realize your own potential for pleasure.

Helping Yourself Become Multi-Orgasmic

Unlike the male orgasm, which has received very little scrutiny, the female orgasm has been the subject of countless volumes over the last century—most written by men, of course. (We discuss this research and its most important findings in the section called "Her Orgasm" in chapter 4.) In the West, much controversy has surrounded the exact nature of the female orgasm—vaginal, clitoral, or a blend of the two. Unfortunately, much of this investigation has really been an attempt to create an "ideal" female orgasm. We believe, along with sexologists Hartman, Fithian, and Campbell, that each woman has an orgasmic pattern that is so individual it can be called her *orgasmic fingerprint*. We also recognize that, even for the same woman, each orgasm has its own specific characteristics, sensations, and levels of satisfaction. (As men move beyond the Big Bang ejaculatory orgasm, they discover that they can have a variety of orgasms, too.)

As far as women's genital orgasms go, the most recent research suggests that there are actually two different nerves involved: the pudendal nerve, which goes to the clitoris; and the pelvic nerve, which goes to the vagina and uterus (see figure 30). The fact that there are two nerves might explain why many women experience clitoral and vaginal orgasms differently. The fact that the two nerves

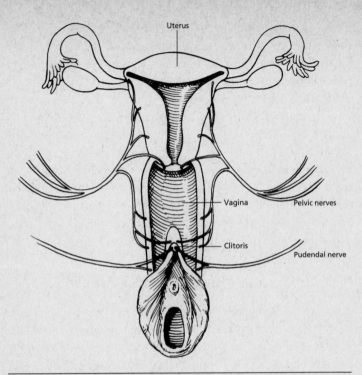

FIGURE 30. PUDENDAL AND PELVIC NERVES

overlap in the spine may also explain why some women experience "blended" orgasms. According to the Tao, genital orgasms—clitoral, vaginal, or blended—are just the beginning. The Taoists have known all along that you can feel orgasmic pulsations and pleasure in any part of your body—your clitoris, your vagina, your brain, even your internal organs.

YOUR CLITORIS

About 70 percent of all women require some clitoral stimulation to have an orgasm, perhaps because the pudendal nerve, which goes to the clitoris, has more nerve endings than the pelvic nerve the vagina. In most lovemaking positions, the man directly stimulates the most sensitive part of his penis, the head, while the woman only indirectly stimulates the most sensitive part of her sexual anatomy, the clitoris.

Encouraging your partner, as we do in this book, to stimulate your clitoris during lovemaking is a clear way to help yourself become more orgasmic. Though it may seem a little awkward at first as he is learning to coordinate the rhythm of his fingers with the rhythm of his hips, it will soon become a smooth and satisfying part of your lovemaking. You can also help him by guiding his hand to where you would like it to be and even using your fingers to press his fingers into your clitoris, which will show him the place and the amount of pressure you like. If you are vaginally orgasmic you may not need or want clitoral stimulation all the time when you are making love. Your hand can guide your partner's, depending on what your pleasure calls for.

Some women are bashful about asking for what they want, but many studies have shown that women who are able to ask for or show their partners what they want will much more often get it. Female sexual passivity and reticence are an outdated holdover from Victorian attitudes. There are few things as arousing to a man as an active and excited partner. Passive and active, according to the Tao, are complementary parts of all sexuality, both male and female.

Sometimes it may be easiest for you to help yourself have an orgasm by squeezing your thighs or directly touching your clitoris during lovemaking. You may be interested to know that although we often think of men as able to reach orgasm much faster than women during intercourse, women have actually been shown to be able to orgasm just as quickly as men when they pleasure themselves. According to a study of multi-orgasmic women conducted by sex researchers at the University of Wisconsin, multi-orgasmic women were more likely to "enhance clitoral stimulation during intercourse by thigh pressure or masturbation."[3] The multi-orgasmic women were also more likely to enjoy having their breasts fondled and their nipples kissed, to give and receive oral sex, to use erotic fantasies, literature, and films, and to have a sensitive partner to whom they could communicate their needs. The study concluded that women don't become multi-orgasmic by accident. They choose the techniques that maximize their pleasure and tell their partners about them.

Many women are ashamed to self-pleasure with their partner or even by themselves. With the amount of stigma surrounding masturbation, this anxiety is quite understandable. If this is an issue for you, please read the section called "Self-Pleasuring and Self-Cultivation" in chapter 3. Here let us just say that self-pleasuring is a healthy and important way of cultivating your sexuality that complements lovemaking and does not replace it. *Human Sexuality,* a book published by the American Medical Association (and mentioned in chapter 3), states that women tend to self-pleasure more as they grow older. The more you take an active role in your pleasure, the more likely you are to reach your full sexual potential. In the wise words of one businesswoman in her late fifties, "In life, everyone is responsible for their own orgasm."

There are two factors that generally influence whether a woman is able to have vaginal or blended orgasms as well as clitoral orgasms: the sensitivity of her G spot or other internal spots, and the strength of her PC muscle.

YOUR G SPOT AND OTHER SENSITIVE SPOTS

You may have heard about a place in your vagina that when touched is supposed to drive you wild. This place is often called the *G spot,* named for physician Ernest Gräfenberg, who first described it in 1950. More recently, it has also been called the *inner trigger point* and the *urethral sponge.* Although the idea of the G spot is not new, it is still controversial, some women finding the G spot and others not. The current theory is that the G spot is a collection of glands, ducts, blood vessels, and nerve endings that surround a woman's urethra.

So where exactly is it? Most women who report finding their G spot describe it as located one and a half to two inches from the opening of their vagina. You can feel it through the upper front wall, just behind your pubic bone (see figure 18 on page 88). If you imagine a clock with your clitoris as twelve o'clock, the G spot is usually somewhere between eleven and one.

When you are not aroused, your G spot is difficult to find. When stimulated, it can swell to the size of a dime or larger, standing out from the wall of the vagina. Alan and Donna Brauer suggest that the best time to find it is just after you have orgasmed: "It is already somewhat enlarged and sensitive. It often feels like little ridges or tiny bumps." They recommend stroking it (or having your partner stroke it) at the rate of about once a second and experimenting with both lighter and heavier pressure. Another good time to stimulate the G spot is when you are just approaching orgasm, since you are more likely to enjoy G-spot stimulation once you are already highly aroused.

You should be aware that some women feel initial discomfort or the urge to urinate when their G spot is stimulated. This is normal. If it happens to you, the Brauers suggest lightening your touch or telling your partner to lighten his. It may take as much as a minute for the discomfort or seeming need to urinate to be replaced with pleasurable sensations. If you are concerned about urinating, you might urinate before lovemaking or try finding the G spot while sitting on the toilet, which will allow you to feel confident that your bladder is empty.

In the common face-to-face or missionary position, your partner's penis often misses your G spot completely. It is easier for your partner to stimulate it if you lie on your stomach and your partner enters you from behind, or if you are on top, where you can position yourself for maximum pleasure. Shallow thrusting is also best for stimulating the G spot. However, fingers (yours or his) are usually the most direct and effective way to get to the G spot at first.

Some women report that their most sensitive spots are located at the four o'clock and eight o'clock positions about midway back along the walls of the vagina. There are nerve bundles at these locations, which may explain their sensitivity to pressure. Other women find that they are most sensitive at the back of their vagina. As your partner learns shallow and deep thrusting in different directions (what we call *screwing*), he will be able to stimulate these spots and others that are all your own.

Most women are able to rotate their pelvis when they are on top to direct their partner's penis to their most sensitive spots. As

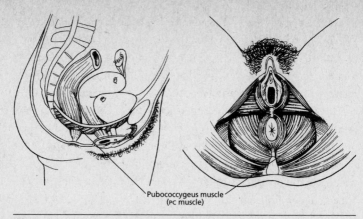

Pubococcygeus muscle
(PC muscle)

FIGURE 31. WOMAN'S PC MUSCLE

we discuss in chapter 5, there are many benefits to this woman-on-top position, and not only for the woman, since many men have an easier time learning to be multi-orgasmic when they are on the bottom. However, this position also has its disadvantages: the angle of penetration in this position can make your partner's penis seem as much as an inch shorter than in other positions, and it is more difficult for your partner to maintain an erection for an extended period of time, since gravity tends to draw blood out of his penis. When women are on the bottom, they often do not realize that they can actively rotate their pelvis, and especially their sacrum, to guide their partner's penis to their most sensitive spots. Once you and your partner learn to rock 'n' roll your pelvises, you will really be "dirty" dancing. (For a longer discussion about various lovemaking positions, see the section called "Positions for Pleasure and Health" in chapter 5.)

YOUR SEX MUSCLE

Your sex muscle, or pubococcygeus muscle (often simply called the PC muscle), is the muscular sling that stretches from your pubic bone in front to your tailbone in back (see figure 31), encircling your urethra, vagina, and anus. It forms a sling that supports not only your uterus, fallopian tubes, and ovaries, but all of your internal organs. If your PC muscle isn't strong, you have no foundation for your organs and they can begin to sag.

Most women will recognize the PC as the muscle they use to stop themselves from urinating when they can't find a toilet. It is also the perineal muscle that must be strong and flexible to avoid tearing during childbirth. Still, the strain of childbirth can weaken your PC muscle. As Senior Healing Tao instructor and acupuncturist Dr. Angela Shen explains, "Especially after a woman has a baby, she has a tendency to get tired more easily and not to enjoy sex as much. Not all women, but many." For these women, Sexual Kung Fu can help them regain their energy and sexual strength.

The importance of the PC muscle was discovered in the West during the 1940s by Arnold Kegel, a gynecologist. He developed the famous Kegel (pronounced *KAY-gul*) exercises, which helped many women control their bladders and ease childbirth. Later, women began to use these exercises to increase their sexual desire, intensify their orgasms, and become multi-orgasmic. Dr. Shen points out: "All women can experience more orgasms and expand the ones they have by doing these practices."

FINDING YOUR PC MUSCLE

The easiest way to find your PC muscle is to stop the flow of urine by clamping down the muscles in your pelvis the next time you are urinating. Make sure you keep your stomach and legs relaxed. You want to try to isolate your PC muscle. If you have a strong PC muscle, you should be able to stop the flow of urine midstream and then start it again. If this is difficult for you and some urine dribbles out during your contraction, your PC muscle is weak. Not to worry: it will quickly strengthen with practice. If you find it easy to stop and start your urine flow, your PC muscle is strong. Nonetheless, you will still expand your sexual pleasure and your overall health by practicing PC exercises.

Strengthening this muscle will not only improve your sex life, but will also help you avoid bladder problems in the future (or improve bladder problems that you may already have). Stopping the flow of urine may sting at first. This is a perfectly normal reaction

PARTNER EXERCISE 1

STOPPING THE STREAM

1. Exhale slowly and forcefully, pushing out the urine.
2. Inhale and contract your PC muscle to stop the flow of urine midstream. (Make sure your stomach and legs are relaxed.)
3. Exhale and start urinating again.
4. Repeat steps 2 and 3 four or five times or until you have finished urinating.

PARTNER EXERCISE 2

PC PULL-UPS

1. Inhale and concentrate on your vagina.
2. As you exhale, contract your PC muscle and the muscles around your eyes and mouth.
3. Inhale and relax, releasing your PC, eye, and mouth muscles.
4. Repeat, contracting your muscles as you exhale and releasing them as you inhale, nine to thirty-six times.

and should stop within a few weeks, unless for some reason you have an infection, in which case you should wait until you have seen a doctor and cleared it up before continuing with the practice. If your muscles become sore, you just need practice.

STRENGTHENING YOUR SEX MUSCLE

There are many different exercises for strengthening your PC muscle that have been taught in the West, most of them adaptations of Kegel's original technique. All of these teach you to contract and relax the PC muscle, although the number of repetitions and the amount of time they suggest you hold the contractions vary widely. The PC Pull-Ups exercise is based on a traditional Taoist technique. It also uses the Taoist awareness that the circular muscles of the body (those in your eyes, mouth, perineum, and anus) are connected. By squeezing the muscles around your eyes and mouth, you can increase the force of your PC Pull-Ups.

Although contracting your eyes and lips will help you squeeze your PC muscle around your vagina, *the most important part of the practice is simply contracting and releasing your PC muscle as often as you can,* which you can do practically anywhere—while driving, while watching TV, while sending a fax, while in a boring meeting. You can see how many contractions you can do during a red light, or you can hold a single contraction until the light turns green. Eventually you will be able to do the contractions with less effort and without contracting your eyes and lips.

Try to do the exercise at least two or three times a day, although you can do it is as many times as you like. Your muscles may get sore, just as they do after you do any exercise. Don't push yourself too far; just increase the repetitions gradually. Consistency is more important than quantity. One way to develop a daily routine is to connect your practice to daily events, like getting up in the morning, taking a shower, or lying in bed at night.

Another, even more effective way to strengthen your PC muscle is to squeeze the muscle against something—your finger, your partner's finger, a vibrator, a dildo, or your partner's penis. The resistance will help you better squeeze the muscle. Try squeezing your fist. You can tighten it only so much, but if you try squeezing your fist around a finger or two of your other hand, you will be able to tighten it even more. The same concept applies to your PC muscle.

If you are practicing with a partner, you can squeeze on your partner's finger or penis and he can tell you how strong your PC muscle is. If you are having intercourse, each of you can alternate squeezing your PC muscles. When you contract yours, you will tighten around his penis and increase sensations for both of you. When he squeezes his, he will raise his erection toward his belly and possibly stimulate your G spot. Another highly enjoyable practice is for you to relax your PC muscle when you thrust together and then tighten your PC muscle when you separate. This will increase the feeling of suction during intercourse and can be very arousing for both of you.

STRENGTHENING YOUR ENTIRE VAGINA

1. Insert a stone egg while standing or sitting. (If you do not feel sufficiently lubricated, you can moisten the egg with water, saliva, or a water-soluble lubricant (for example, K-Y jelly).

2. Contract your PC muscle to pull the egg into your vagina and then bear down slightly and push the egg out toward the opening of your vagina.

3. Repeat this in-and-out movement nine, eighteen, or thirty-six times.

4. When you are done, bear down more forcefully and expel your egg.

STRENGTHENING YOUR ENTIRE VAGINA

In China, women used a special egg-shaped stone to strengthen their PC and other vaginal muscles. We have found jade stone, shaped like an egg, to be best. Doing PC Pull-Ups will certainly strengthen your PC muscle considerably, but you can accelerate the process dramatically by using a stone egg for resistance. In the West, physicians are now prescribing exercises with stainless-steel weights, called *weighted tampons,* to strengthen women's pelvic muscles, especially for women who have trouble controlling their bladder, often after childbirth.[4] But childbirth and pelvic health are not the only reasons to do the egg practice. Women who are knowledgeable in the Tao have used this practice for millennia to increase their vaginal-muscle control for increasing their and their partner's sexual pleasure.

The egg practice is quite simple. You insert a lubricated egg into your vagina (as you would a tampon) and then use your vaginal muscles to move it up and down. Once the egg is deeper inside, you may not feel it at all, but you can continue moving the egg up and down by squeezing your perineum and vagina to move the egg up and then bearing down slightly (as you would to have a bowel movement) to move the egg back down (see figure 32). Then you can squeeze your perineum and vagina to push it up once again

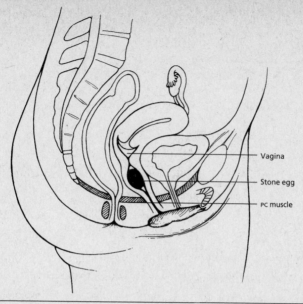

FIGURE 32. STONE-EGG EXERCISE

and then push it back down. You can do this exercise for two minutes and then, bearing down more forcefully, expel the egg.

Senior Healing Tao instructor Marcia Kerwit explains how to
prepare and take care of your stone egg: "When you get your egg
home, you first want to sterilize it, which you can do by boiling it
for ten minutes or soaking it in a solution of one part household
bleach to ten parts of water for ten minutes. Rinse it well. You
need to sterilize your egg only the first time you use it. After that,
you can rinse it off with soap and water after each use, or just soak
it in a vinegar solution."

You can order a drilled jade egg from the Healing Tao Center
(see the appendix), which will allow you to loop dental floss through
your egg and leave the floss hanging outside your vagina, so that
after practicing you can pull it out easily, just like a tampon. One ad-
vantage of using the drilled egg with the dental-floss tail is that as
you move your egg up and down in your vagina, you can feel the
string moving as well, so you will feel that it is actually moving and
how far. (You will find more details about the egg exercise and other

Sexual Kung Fu exercises for women in *Healing Love Through the Tao: Cultivating Female Sexual Energy;* see appendix.)

What If . . .

MY EGG IS STUCK

If you use an egg *without* a string, it may occasionally feel like it's stuck. If this happens, the most important thing is not to panic. Remember, the egg can't go very far. Calmly, see if your vagina feels dry inside. If so, you can use your finger to put some more (water-based) lubricant in your vagina and around the opening. Try squatting down or sitting on the toilet and bearing down to push the egg out. If the egg still does not come out, you can try jumping up and down and laughing. Then try squatting and bearing down again. If the egg still has not come out, go do something else. During this time, your muscles will relax and the egg will most likely move on its own and be easier to expel. Finally, you can insert your finger (or, more easily, a friend or partner can insert one) and direct the egg out. This should allow you to get the egg out, but if you are still having a problem, call a Healing Tao instructor. If you use a drilled egg that has string looped through it, you will never have this problem.

MY EGG SMELLS FUNNY WHEN I TAKE IT OUT

An unusual smell to your secretions could indicate a vaginal infection. This has nothing to do with using the egg, but you should not do the egg exercises (or the Big Draw) until the infection is gone. There are many simple home remedies for vaginal infections. Speak to someone at a women's clinic or to a health practitioner.

You may find that doing these exercises and strengthening your PC muscle in general can cause you to become sexually aroused. The reason to develop your PC muscle in the first place is to reach your orgasmic potential, and if your partner is a multi-orgasmic man, you should have no problem satisfying your increased desire. If you do not have a partner or your partner is not around, you can either pleasure yourself or use the Big Draw exercise described later in this chapter to move your sexual energy away from your genitals and to the rest of your body, where it will energize and rejuvenate you.

DEEP VAGINAL AND UTERINE ORGASMS

As we mentioned earlier, women have two different genital nerves: the pudendal, which connects to the clitoris and surrounding skin; and the pelvic, which connects to the vagina and the uterus. With some awareness and a little practice women can experience deep vaginal and uterine contractions. One multi-orgasmic woman described her experience: "First, I practiced by myself. I would tighten and release my vaginal muscles and then move these contractions up toward my uterus. Soon, the contractions would begin involuntarily during lovemaking. They were truly incredible."

These extremely pleasurable and powerful orgasms were well known in China to women who practiced the Tao and who were able to control their vaginal and uterine muscles through the egg practice. In the 1980s the Brauers studied these deep pelvic "push-out" contractions, which they called "extended sexual response." They even noticed from electrical brain recordings (EEGs) that a woman's brain waves during these uterine orgasms seemed to resemble those observed in people who are in deep meditation. The Taoists have always taught women that they can help themselves experience these profound orgasms by developing their awareness of and connection to their deep vaginal and uterine muscles.

CIRCULATING SEXUAL ENERGY

If you learn to circulate energy yourself, you will be able to expand your orgasms throughout your body. Dr. Angela Shen explains: "If you draw energy up before and during your orgasm it

DEEPENING YOUR ORGASMS

1. Picture what your uterus looks like (see figure 33). When you are able to envision a part of your body, you are able to make a stronger connection to it, linking your mind and your body.

2. Next find out where *your* uterus is located. Stand and place your thumbs together at your navel and make a triangle with your index fingers (see figure 34). Where your index fingers touch is approximately the level of your uterus. Your uterus is the size of a small plum. (Where your little fingers naturally fall is approximately where your ovaries are.)

3. Inhale, and as you exhale contract your eyes and your mouth lightly and feel the back of your vagina deep inside you contracting (where your cervix is). When you do this correctly, you will have a light orgasmic feeling deep inside you.

will be more intense and last longer. You will also be less tired afterward." Circulating sexual energy brings healing energy to your entire body and allows you and your partner to have truly ecstatic lovemaking. This ability to circulate sexual energy is the basis for both transcendent sexuality and vibrant health. (If you ejaculate it is even more important that you practice conserving and circulating this energy, because otherwise you will become drained.[5])

The Big Draw for Women exercise on page 168 will help you circulate your sexual energy through your body. Many women are able to start drawing the energy up without much practice. As one multi-orgasmic man recalls, "Without having had any meditation practice or experience, my girlfriend was able to draw up the energy in her body instinctively, as apparently many women are."

Overcoming Difficulty

As we discuss in the section called "Brain Waves and Reflexes" in chapter 1, Western science has recently confirmed that orgasm is as much a state of mind as a state of body. And the state of your

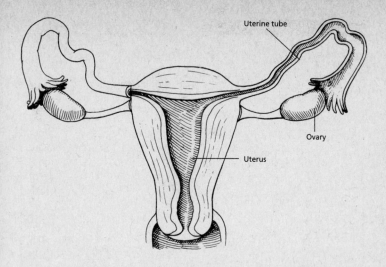

FIGURE 33. THE UTERUS

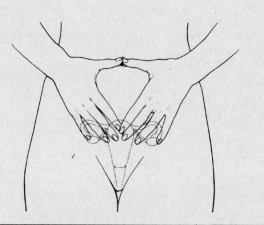

FIGURE 34. LOCATING YOUR UTERUS

mind has much to do with what you learn. Back in 1939, anthro-
pologist Margaret Mead demonstrated how much orgasm is dependent on cultural expectations. She compared two neighboring
peoples living on the Pacific island of New Guinea. The Mundugumor believed that women have orgasms, whereas their neighbors

THE BIG DRAW FOR WOMEN

1. Picture your vagina and clitoris. If you don't know what they look like, use a mirror and have a look.

2. Lightly touch the lips of your vagina and your clitoris until you are starting to get aroused.

3. Inhale, and as you exhale, lightly contract your vagina, squeezing around your clitoris.

4. Inhale and release, imagining your vagina expanding like a flower blossoming.

5. Repeat exhaling and contracting, then inhaling and releasing, nine to thirty-six times.

6. Imagine your uterus and ovaries also opening and closing like flowers blossoming.

7. When you feel your sexual energy expanding, relax and bring the energy to your tailbone and sacrum and then up your spine to your brain (see figure 35). Or if you are having difficulty bringing the energy up, try contracting your vagina and your anus as you direct the orgasmic feeling back to your tailbone and sacrum and then up the spine to your brain. (If you still do not feel your energy moving up, you may want to try activating your sacral and cranial pumps, as we describe in chapter 3.)

8. Let the orgasmic energy flow down through the rest of your body or direct it to any part of your body that needs healing or strengthening.

the Arapash did not. Not surprisingly, most Mundugumor women were orgasmic, whereas most Arapash women were not.[6] Given the importance of cultural permission for pleasure, many women around the globe and throughout history have had their orgasmic potential limited by societal expectations.

Women generally have one of two kinds of orgasmic problems. If you have never had an orgasm, you are *preorgasmic*. If you orgasm on some occasions but not others, by yourself but not with a partner, or with some partners but not others, you are *situationally orgasmic*. Almost all women who are preorgasmic can learn to have orgasms fairly easily. The most important factor is a willingness to

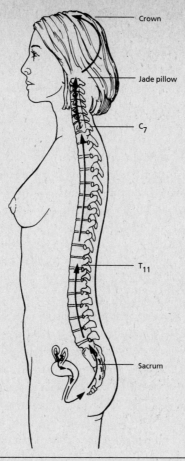

FIGURE 35. DRAWING SEXUAL ENERGY UP

learn to pleasure yourself and to take charge of your pleasure during lovemaking. First, of course, you must be willing to stimulate yourself. (If this is difficult for you, see the discussion earlier in this chapter and in the section called "Self-Pleasuring and Self-Cultivation" in chapter 3.)

First, you need to begin by getting acquainted with your body and your sexuality. Negative feelings about your body or how you look during lovemaking can distract you and short-circuit your ability to experience pleasure and have an orgasm. Start by taking a noncritical look at yourself in the mirror. Appreciate your body for its beauty and its ability to give you pleasure. Then start to explore your body. Be sure to stroke your entire body before focusing on your genitals. You may want to use oil, which can magnify the stimulation. Sex therapists are fond of pointing out that your brain is your most important sex organ, so be sure to put yourself into an erotic frame of mind. You may wish to remember a particularly satisfying experience of lovemaking, to read erotica, or to create a fantasy out of your own imagination's rich storehouse of fantasies and desires.

According to both Kinsey and Hite, four out of five women who self-pleasure rely on clitoral stimulation to experience an orgasm. The type of clitoral stroke depends on you: hard or soft, stimulation of the shaft or head, up and down, side to side, or circular touch. Experiment and see what you find pleasurable. You may also find that a vibrator can help you reach orgasm. Find one that you like. Almost all women can learn to orgasm through self-pleasuring. Remember that all orgasms are not the same. Many orgasmic women think they are not so because they expect their orgasm to match someone else's pattern or to involve the earth moving and the stars tumbling down. According to Lonnie Barbach, "Most women's initial experience of orgasm is mild, while their expectations reflect the proverbial fireworks."[7] She adds that vaginal orgasms can be very diffuse and tame while clitoral orgasms tend to be more discrete and recognizable.

When you are ready to "go public," let your partner stimulate you in the ways you have found you enjoy. Make sure to tell him what you like or to show him. When you are ready, try intercourse. Remember that you can take responsibility for your own pleasure. Position yourself where you find the best stimulation and continue to touch yourself or guide your partner's hand to your clitoris. During intercourse, guide your partner's penis with your pelvis to where you feel the greatest stimulation.

If you have had orgasms at some point in your life but no longer do, you need to determine what has changed. Is your health different? Are you suffering from an infection or taking medication that might decrease your arousal? Many women experience reduced arousal during pregnancy or while breast-feeding, although others do not. If you think the problem is physical, consult a physician. Certain drugs and certain conditions, such as diabetes, can inhibit orgasm. Has your partner changed? Or has your relationship changed in some way? Do you have feelings of anger or resentment that you are not expressing? Are you distracted by children or work? It is important to address any or all of these situations before you work on expanding your pleasure.

If you are orgasmic when self-pleasuring but not when making love, you may need to determine what you are not getting with your partner. Are you too focused on his pleasure? Are you too self-conscious? Are you not getting fully aroused? Try extending foreplay and making sure that you are totally aroused before intercourse, or forget about intercourse for the time being and focus on pleasuring each other with your hands and mouths. Orgasming before you have intercourse also will make it easier for you to orgasm when you are having intercourse.

If you are able to experience orgasm through manual or oral loving but not through intercourse, are you experiencing pain during intercourse? If so, are you lubricated enough? Are you able to choose the angle and amount of thrusting? If not, try another position. If pain is not the problem but you are still not orgasmic during intercourse, have your partner use his hands or mouth to bring you to orgasm before you engage in a coital embrace. Also explore or let your partner explore your G spot or other sensitive spots. Try the positions—you on top, rear entry, sitting in his lap—that tend to stimulate the G spot most. And remember to use your trusty fingers, with or without his, to reach orgasm.

If you are still unable to have an orgasm, do not despair. There are lots of resources for preorgasmic women, including books, groups, and counseling. In addition, you should know that with Taoist sexuality you can experience extremely high levels of pleasure throughout your entire body whether you have orgasms or not. Learning to circulate sexual energy and pleasure throughout your body will allow you to experience a fusion of energy with yourself and your partner that makes the "Did you or didn't you?" question largely irrelevant. More important than reaching orgasm or becoming multi-orgasmic is learning to experience the heights of pleasure and intimacy that come from the true union of body, heart, mind, and spirit.

CHAPTER SEVEN

Yang and Yang

For Gay Men

China, like all civilizations, has long acknowledged the practice of homosexuality. Historically it was called *lung-yang,* after the name of a fourth-century B.C. prince's male lover, or *tuan-hsiu,* "the cut sleeve," recalling an emperor who was said to have cut off his sleeve to avoid waking his sleeping lover.[1] Although sexual relationships between men were at times condoned and at other times discouraged by the imperial court—no doubt depending on who was sleeping in the royal bed—Taoism has never condemned homosexuality. Taoism avoids condemning any part of human sexual experience, since it is all considered a part of the Tao. Rather, Taoism tries to teach people how to stay healthy, whatever their sexual preferences. Gay men simply need to know the practices that will help them have satisfying and healthy sexual relationships.

Can't Stop Till I Get Enough

A gay writer and activist was doing a radio interview about his book on life in the pre-AIDS bathhouses, where gay men often would have numerous sexual encounters per night. When asked about whether the desire for multiple sexual experiences is characteristic of gay men in general, the author shot back that it is characteristic of all male sexuality, but that straight men are usually constrained by female sexuality. If, he continued, we really want to see what male sexuality is like, uninfluenced by female sexuality, we just need to look at gay men.

The Taoist understands this characteristic of male sexuality in terms of the properties of masculine energy, or yang (see chapter 5 for an explanation of yin and yang). Yang is active, volatile, and expansive. During heterosexual sex, the woman's yin receives and balances the man's yang. (As we mentioned in chapter 5, yin and yang are variable qualities that exist in both men and women. There are some men who are more yin and some women who are more yang. According to the Taoists the universe always seeks balance in relationships as in nature.)

In general, when two gay men make love, each man's yang charges the other's, increasing rather than diminishing their sexual desire. Gay Healing Tao instructor B. J. Santerre explains the value of multiple orgasms for gay men: "Gay men really need multiple orgasms. Most straight men are going to do it once or twice in an evening. For gay men it's really common that they need more than that in a night. With this practice you are going to be able to fully satisfy this desire whether you have a partner or not."

The expansiveness of yang energy is hard to contain and often will want to escape through the most direct route—the penis. It is no surprise that the object of much gay male sexuality, according to gay sex educator and healer Joseph Kramer, is "to get it up and off." This emphasis on ejaculation is understandable because it allows you to satisfy your sexual desire; once a man ejaculates he becomes more yin—in other words, stable, internal, and contractive.

To avoid this endless cycle of ejaculation, which is extremely depleting to your body and your immune system, you need to cultivate your own yin energy and to spread your expanding yang energy throughout your body. Channeling this energy and containing it is also, as we explained earlier, the way to become multi-orgasmic and to experience whole-body orgasms that will be more satisfying than the genital "getting off" that most men are accustomed to. As B. J. Santerre explains, "If you conserve your semen, you are going to be able to go back to the heydays when people would go to the bathhouses and have orgasms all night long. When you learn this practice, you are able to do the same thing, but you won't exhaust yourself and you won't even need to leave home!"

Cultivating Your Sexual Energy

Gay men, like all men, need to learn to circulate their sexual energy though their body both to expand their orgasms and to benefit from the power and healing potential of their sexual energy. During nonejaculatory sex, it is even more important for men to draw this energy up in order to satisfy their desire and transform the volatile sexual energy (*ching-chi*) into the more refined and stable *chi*. We discussed the techniques for circulating your sexual energy and for separating orgasm from ejaculation in chapters 2 and 3. Here we just want to describe the importance of these practices for gay men and gay male couples.

One multi-orgasmic gay man described his experience: "I had a lover in New York, and I was so much into the Tao, I said, 'You have to get into it.' I didn't give him a choice. When we felt like fooling around, we'd start playing with one another. When each of us would feel ready we would do the Big Draw at our own speed. When we did it together, even if we didn't circulate the energy at the same time, we would be satisfied at the same point. We would fall asleep in two minutes. That sharing of energy keeps going on as you sleep in one another's arms, because you are both charged with sexual energy."

As we said in chapter 3, these practices can be done on your own or even if your partner is not "into the Tao." As one multi-orgasmic gay man explained, "After pleasing myself or making love and doing the Big Draw four or five times, I am done. After that if the most gorgeous guy is right in front of me and he says, 'Let me suck you off,' I'll say, 'Please, leave me alone.' I'm satisfied even though I haven't ejaculated."

If you find you are having difficulty controlling your yang sexual energy, you may be in need of some balancing and calming yin energy. Fortunately, there are many sources of yin energy, since both yin and yang exist in all of nature, from the cosmic (earth and heaven) to the microcosmic (your body). Since each of us has both yin and yang, you can cultivate within yourself the qualities of yin such as gentleness, kindness, and self-respect. (For a fuller discussion of learning how to cultivate these qualities and how to deal with emotional imbalances, see Mantak Chia's *Taoist Ways to Transform Stress into Vitality*.) From the environment, you can balance your energy by eating yin foods such as vegetables and fish or by absorbing yin energy directly from the earth. According to Taoism (as well as many other traditions), the earth is feminine (that is, yin). Men can absorb yin energy from the earth simply through spending time in nature and gardening or can absorb it in a more concentrated form by drawing energy up from the earth when practicing the Cool Draw, described in chapter 3.

Being Versatile

Most gay men are aware of the pleasure potential of their prostate and their anus (if you are not, see "Prostate" in chapter 2). Yet some gay men still disparage men who are "bottoms." This attitude is not surprising given the negative stigma associated with "getting fucked" and the links in Western society between power and being on top. As we mentioned in chapter 5 in regard to heterosexual couples, Taoism sees the person on top not as dominating but as healing his or her partner. The person on top (or the more active partner) gives more sexual energy (and healing) to the person on the bottom (or the more passive partner).

According to the Tao, everything that is active must also be passive, and therefore it is recommended that gay men be versatile—both "tops" and "bottoms." As one multi-orgasmic man explained, the sexual benefits are obvious: "A guy who has been both a top and a bottom is a great lover because he knows what it is like to satisfy his partner and to be satisfied. If you are only a top, you know only one version. The same if you are a bottom."

When you are the bottom, you also have the benefit of having your prostate massaged during anal intercourse. According to Stephen T. Chang in his book *The Tao of Sexology,* gay men who generally are bottoms have far fewer prostate problems than tops and heterosexual men.[2] Nevertheless, most men have their preference and may not want to experiment.

If you are a top who is not willing to be a bottom, you can still benefit from having your anus stimulated and from exercising your anal-sphincter muscle. B. J. Santerre explains: "When people think about penetration, everybody just thinks about a big ten-inch dick or a dildo, but it can be a small finger. Being penetrated needs some practice, like everything else. You need the proper partner to take it easy, and you need to relax those muscles. It's not on the first day that you are going to get fucked. And if you don't like to be penetrated, you can still play with your anus. Even stimulating the outside of the anus is very important because you can strengthen your butt muscles, which are essential for circulating the sexual energy."

It is also worth mentioning that bottoms can be active as well as passive. The more you exercise your PC muscle (see chapter 3) and your anal sphincter, the more you can massage your partner's penis and pleasure both of you. B. J. Santerre continues: "If your anus is really strong, you are going to be a great fuck for your partner. You are going to massage his penis as he is penetrating you. You are not totally passive and just waiting for it to happen. You take part in it by contracting and releasing the lower part or the higher part. You can contract it really fast two or three times in a row or just let your partner get a little bit deeper and surprise him by squeezing it."

Gay and straight men who are just beginning to experiment with anal stimulation sometimes worry that they may tear the skin of the anus or the colon. The solution here is simply to use enough lubrication and to have a gentle partner. Other gay men worry whether repeated anal sex will weaken their anal sphincter. There is no evidence to suggest that this is the case, and anal sex may in fact strengthen the muscles of your anus. Nonetheless, if you are concerned or feel that your anal muscles are weak, you can try the sphincter exercise given in chapter 9 to strengthen them.

Monogamy and Multiple Partners

The age of AIDS has fostered a new ethic of monogamy for gay men (as well as heterosexuals). Assuming you are using safer-sex techniques, however, there is nothing inherently wrong with multiple partners. The Taoist texts actually instructed heterosexual men about the benefits of a number of partners. But there is a challenge with multiple partners: the practices given in this book require a profound connection of body, heart, mind, and spirit, which is difficult to achieve with even one partner, let alone many. According to the Tao, one profound sexual union, gay or straight, is better than countless superficial ones.

The anonymous sex that has characterized much Western sexuality is diametrically opposed to the kind of physical, emotional, and spiritual connection that Sexual Kung Fu facilitates and requires. Whether you are exchanging bodily fluids or not, you are always exchanging energy. So choose a partner (or partners) wisely.

Safer Sex

Most gay men are highly aware of the need for safer sex and are well informed about the specifics of safer-sex techniques, so we will not discuss the subject at length here. (Should you want more detail about the art and science of condom use and other tricks of the safer-sex trade, see the section called "When to Start: A Few Words About Safer Sex" in chapter 5.) Suffice it to say that we strongly recommend safer sex and that in fact the kind of nonejaculatory sex advocated by the Tao has obvious benefits for reducing the exchange of bodily fluids.

With nonejaculation, not only do you decrease the outflow, you also decrease the inflow. As we mentioned in chapter 5, when you pump out your semen, you create a low-pressure vacuum that draws in liquid or anything else in the environment, such as bacteria or viruses (just as a turkey baster draws up gravy when you squeeze out the air). So when you don't ejaculate, you run less of a risk of drawing in bacteria or viruses. (As you can imagine, this is especially important for anal sex, since the colon naturally has a great many bacteria.)

Bear in mind that even when you practice Sexual Kung Fu, a small amount of ejaculate is often emitted, so you should not forgo other safer-sex precautions.

Sexual Healing

Most people do not understand the healing potential of sexuality. The Taoists have always recognized that sex can both hurt and heal us. Genital sexuality that culminates in ejaculation is draining to the body. As Joseph Kramer has pointed out, we build up life-giving sexual energy in our groin, but instead of bringing this energy up to our brain and heart, where it can begin to help heal us, we clamp down by tightening our chest muscles and holding our breath. With nowhere to go, this energy is stuck in our groin and eventually becomes too great to be contained and forces its way out of our penis as we ejaculate.

In Sexual Kung Fu, you stay very close to the point of no return and even feel the orgasmic contractions, but you do not ejaculate. You do this by learning about your arousal rate, using the techniques described in chapter 3, and, most important, drawing the energy away from your genitals up through your spine and the rest of your body.

Once you have built up this energy, you can also exchange it with your partner. This energy exchange profoundly affects the health and well-being of both partners and takes place even through the walls of latex that we now must necessarily put between us. It is only our Western isolation and individualism that wrongly lead us to believe we can engage in sex without this intimacy and interpenetration. But if we look at the very definition of the word *intercourse*, we find its meaning to be very close to the Taoist understanding: "connection," "exchange," "communion."

Unfortunately, instead of using the appropriate yardstick for sex, which is health, we in the West have used a moral measure. This approach has led us to size up sex according to criteria such as pleasure/pain and purity/perversity, depending on the censors' own predilections. Over the centuries, gay sex, along with much other sexuality, including self-pleasuring, has been defined as perverse, sinful, sick, and unnatural. Saint Augustine and Thomas Aquinas went so far as to call all sexuality that does not lead to conception unnatural.

Because the Taoists were able to see in sex a powerful source of the body's life-sustaining energy, *chi,* they were able to recognize its importance to the overall health of our body, our emotions, our mind, and our spirit. Since the 1980s, we have been tragically reminded of sex's ability to bring illness, but in our frenzy of fear we have forgotten sex's ability to make us well.

Cultivating your sexual energy is therefore especially important if you are living with HIV or AIDS. Many people who are confronting life-threatening illnesses lose their appetite for sex. But this is the very time when they need their sexual energy the most. B. J. Santerre, who has been living with HIV for eleven years, explains: "Sexual energy is so important for the flow of energy in the body that you cannot afford to not use it. Waking up with an erection is an important sign of vitality that many men who are sick no longer experience. When you wake up with a hard-on, you will know your health is improving."

For men (and women) who are sick with AIDS or other sexually transmitted diseases, there are often two additional resistances to utilizing the healing power of sexuality: guilt ("I got it through sex") and fear ("I don't want to get others sick"). These feelings are understandable but misguided. Similarly, having gotten sick through sex doesn't mean you don't need the healing power of your sexuality. People who get sick through the air or from food do not stop breathing or eating. If you are afraid of getting others sick, you can take comfort in the fact that nonejaculatory sex, as we mentioned earlier, makes safer sex even safer. If you remain concerned, you can still do the solo Sexual Kung Fu described in chapters 2 and 3.

It goes without saying that according to the Tao, it is all the more important to conserve your semen when you are confronting a life-threatening disease or any serious sexual illness. As B. J. Santerre explained, "We don't have a cure for AIDS yet, but we do know that some people die right away and others live a long time. When your body is having to make new sperm, it is not going to be making white blood cells."

When you are using Sexual Kung Fu to help heal serious illness, it is essential that you give your body time to "digest" this growing energy. As one multi-orgasmic man, who had overcome a serious health problem, explained, "The sexual energy is very healing, but this healing process is a lot of work for your body. It can even be uncomfortable in the beginning. Old symptoms may come back." Develop your practice slowly as you learn to work with this powerful healing force within your body. In addition to Sexual Kung Fu, you can gain great benefit from the other Taoist healing arts. (See the appendix for a listing of additional Healing Tao books and resources.)

CHAPTER EIGHT

Before You Call the Plumber

At some point in our lives, most of us experience some kind of sexual problem. You may find yourself ejaculating quickly with a new partner or having difficulty getting an erection with an old one. It is most important to recognize that these are temporary frustrations that reflect the different seasons of our lives and relationships.

In the West, we have a tendency to get fixated on often unhelpful labels like *premature ejaculation* and *impotence,* which cripple a man's self-esteem and his ability to deal with the changes in his sexuality in an easy, relaxed, and even lighthearted way. A sense of humor is often the best antidote to the overly serious way in which we deal with "sexual problems." The biggest danger, as Masters and Johnson and other sex therapists have pointed out, is getting caught in the cycle of "fear-failure-shame-fear" that often causes these difficulties to take up residence in our bedroom. So, even if you are not currently troubled by one of the following concerns, it is a good idea to read this section so that you will know what to expect and how to deal with these unwelcome guests should they someday crash the party.

It's Not Over Till It's Over: Ending Premature Ejaculation

According to Taoist sexuality, there is really no such thing as "premature ejaculation." We don't say this to put sex therapists and sex surrogates out of business, or to deny that many men ejaculate too soon to satisfy their partners, or for that matter themselves. The point is simply that from the Taoist standpoint, the vast majority of men ejaculate "prematurely." According to Sexual Kung Fu, you should be able to choose when you want to ejaculate, so any unwanted ejaculation is premature. Moreover, if ejaculation is no longer the goal, and you can have orgasms without ejaculation, then most ejaculations are by definition premature, or at least superfluous.

So the question is not whether you can last for a certain number of minutes on the stopwatch but whether you and your partner are satisfied with the duration of your lovemaking. If you practice the exercises in chapter 3, you will learn to postpone your ejaculation for as long as you and your partner wish.

If the problem persists or is especially troublesome, you might want to seek professional help. A sex therapist or sex surrogate will help you figure out if there are deeper psychological reasons you are ejaculating quickly (for example, fear of "getting caught," fear of losing your erection, and so on). A professional may give you a series of exercises with which you can build up your sexual confidence. Following is an example of a sequence of exercises that will help you build your staying power. They are based on the understanding that you must learn to detect, and eventually control, your arousal rate.

LEARNING CONTROL

First, you should have your partner stimulate you manually while you focus on the sensations in your genitals and on stopping as you get close to ejaculating. Once you feel confident of your ability to detect and postpone your ejaculation, you can try intercourse with the woman on top, so that you can continue to focus on your sensations. Next you can try intercourse in different positions, and finally you can try slowing down instead of stopping. You also may want to avoid being on top, since the blood that gravity draws into your penis makes it more difficult for you to maintain control.

It is also best to be with a partner whom you know well and with whom there is no performance pressure. It is also good if your partner can encourage you and help you stay aware of your arousal rate ("That's great," "Nice and slow," "Relax"). Your partner also can learn how to move her hips and sacrum to rub your penis in different directions while you stay still. If your partner can learn this practice, you will both experience very high orgasmic levels without ejaculating.

Bear in mind that almost all young men are relatively quick ejaculators, and as men get older they generally have an easier time lasting longer. Also, as you may have noticed in your experience, the longer it's been since you had sex, the more difficult it is to control the ejaculatory urge. Therefore, the more you have sex, the easier it is to control your ejaculation. As we mentioned in the last section on safer sex, condoms can also help men diminish some of the sensitivity in their penis.

LEARNING SEXUAL SENSITIVITY

Many men think that a few drinks might distract them from their pleasure and help delay ejaculation. As one multi-orgasmic man recalls, "One of the things I used to do, and I think a lot of guys have learned to do, is to have a few drinks before you go to bed and suddenly you are not very connected with your groin and you can make love longer because it is harder to have an orgasm because you're buzzed and you are not really there. But it was very frustrating because I would usually ejaculate anyway." It may seem like ejaculating too quickly is the result of too much genital sensitivity, but in fact it is the result of too little. Alcohol is an anesthetic and therefore numbs sensation. Though alcohol may dampen your arousal, it also diminishes your ability to control it. The key to developing real, lasting control is more sensitivity, not less. For this reason baseball statistics also don't work. In addition, it is much more difficult to be aware of your partner's needs when you are drunk or trying to remember Pete Rose's batting average.

Alcohol can also cause the other major male sexual complaint—impotence, or the inability to get an erection, sometimes called *whiskey dick*. Marijuana also has its sexual drawbacks if used regularly. Daily marijuana use has been found to lower androgens, which are directly responsible for your sex drive. This effect can cause decreased interest in sex and difficulty in getting erections. Other studies have shown that repeated use of marijuana can lower your sperm count. Prolonged lovemaking and multiple orgasms have been shown to increase the levels of your body's natural pleasure drug, endorphin. You are much better off skipping the social lubricants in favor of sexual lubricants. Not to mention, endorphins don't give you a hangover.

Snake Charming: Overcoming Impotence

The Yellow Emperor said, "I want to have intercourse but my penis will not rise. I feel so embarrassed that my perspiration comes out like pearls. In my heart I crave to make love and I wish I could help with my hands. How can I help? I wish to hear the Tao." Su Nü replied, "Your Majesty's problem is a problem of all men."[1]

At some point in their sexual lives, all men have the experience of not being able to get an erection or of losing the one they have. The machinery is too complex to be foolproof, but most of the time there is little to worry about. Physical stress (exhaustion, a cold, intoxication) or emotional stress (adjusting to a new partner, performance anxiety, tension in the relationship) can cause your penis to remain limp or to shrink at an inopportune moment. The most important thing to remember at these troubling times is that it is best to take the situation in stride, with a sense of humor and without blaming yourself or your partner. It does not mean that you are any less of a man or that your partner is any less of a woman. Su Nü's first suggestion to the Yellow Emperor was to relax and try to harmonize with his partner.

EXERCISE 14

SOFT ENTRY

1. Your partner must be fully lubricated, and you should pleasure her until her fluids are flowing. If necessary, you can use a lubricant on her vagina or your penis or both.

2. It is generally easiest for you to be on top so that gravity helps draw the blood into your penis and so that you have as much freedom to move as possible.

3. Circle your thumb and forefinger around the base of your penis to form a finger ring and squeeze gently to push the blood into the shaft and head.

4. Carefully insert your penis into your partner and begin thrusting, keeping your finger ring around the base of your penis.

5. Focus on the blood and sexual energy that are filling your penis and concentrate on the sensations in your penis. Squeeze your perineum and buttocks to push blood into your genitals.

6. Your partner can help stimulate you by playing with your testicles, perineum, and anus.

7. Adjust the tightness of your finger ring to keep your penis engorged enough for thrusting and then remove your fingers when your penis is sufficiently erect for continued thrusting.

8. Reapply the finger ring if your erection wanes (although you generally won't need to do so).

ENTER SOFT, EXIT HARD

Recognizing that all men experience situational impotence at some time or another, the Taoists developed a fail-safe technique they called Soft Entry. The Taoists realized that a man could *help with his hands*, just as the Yellow Emperor had wished. With this technique and with the cooperation of your partner, you can enter your partner even when you are completely flaccid. Once you are inside your partner, the warmth and sensation of lovemaking will allow you to get an erection in short order. The Soft Entry technique dispels the old belief that a man must have a steel-hard erection before having intercourse, and it is a useful part of any man's sexual repertoire. Knowing that you have mastered this technique and can use it when necessary will give you greater confidence when faced with the awkward, but common, situation of a penis that is slow to rise.

CAUSE FOR CONCERN

If you tend to have erection problems every time you make love, you may be one of the 22 million men in America who have a more serious erection problem. First, you should make sure a physiological cause can be ruled out. Diabetes, prostate surgery, hardening of the arteries, alcoholism, spinal-cord injuries, and back problems, among other things, can cause impotence. Medications such as tranquilizers, antidepressants, and antihypertensives (for high blood pressure) can also cause impotence. In the 1950s, few cases of impotence (about 10 percent) were believed to have an organic source, but most urologists now believe that as many as half of all cases, and more in older patients, have some biological basis.[2] (Bear in mind that urologists have a vested interest in cases having a biological basis, since that's what they know how to treat and what they get paid to do.) To see if this is your problem, you can do a little self-diagnosis.

While sleeping at night, most men have at least one or two erections, each lasting about a half hour. First, try to recall whether you have awakened in the last week or two with a medium to hard erection. If so, you probably do not have a physiological condition. If you can't remember, there is a simple test you can do at home. Before going to sleep, lick a strip of postage stamps and attach them in a ring around the base of your limp penis. If, upon awakening, the ring is broken, you are physically capable of getting erections. If the ring is unbroken and you are unable to get an erection through solo cultivation, you should see your doctor.[3]

Even if you do have an organic condition, you should remember that this need not stop you from practicing Sexual Kung Fu. Just as orgasm and ejaculation are separate, so too are erection and orgasm. Hartman and Fithian tell the story of an older couple who had a very happy sex life throughout their marriage, although the man was completely impotent as a result of diabetes. Though he and his wife relied on oral and manual lovemaking, both of them were multi-orgasmic. As you learn to expand your orgasms through-out your whole body, your genital erections and genital orgasms will no longer be the alpha and omega of your sexual life.

GETTING AN ERECTION

Perhaps because our model of male sexuality is based on the experiences of eighteen-year-old men, who tend to get hard quickly and frequently, we think in terms of having a hard-on or not, of being fully erect or not. In reality, there are a number of stages of erection and a number of changes that our penises undergo in becoming erect. As we mentioned in chapter 2, the Taoists noticed that there are actually four stages of erection, or four *attainments*, as they called them: firmness (also referred to as *lengthening*), swelling, hardness, and heat.

A common reason for erection trouble is mechanical—not getting enough stimulation of your genitals. Most men need their penises directly touched, rubbed, or massaged to get hard, and this need increases as men get older. Since women often prefer to have their genitals approached slowly and in ever-smaller circles of touch, they think that men do too. Most men, however, prefer quick and direct stimulation. (Don't forget, this is how most men learn to masturbate.)

Your partner should take a very active role in directly stimulating your genitals with her hands and mouth. Tell your partner what you need and how it feels. You should also be willing to use your hands to help yourself get or keep an erection.

Some men, however, find that too much focus on them and their genitals results in pressure to get an erection. It may help for you and your partner to recognize that soft penises have as many nerve endings as hard penises and can be extremely pleasurable. Certain kinds of touch, especially of the testicles, can be highly pleasurable without leading to an erection. Let your partner know that she can pleasure you even if you don't get hard right away. If you find that focusing on your genitals only makes you more anxious, switch the focus to your partner, which was Su Nü's second suggestion. Taking a detour from the man's erection and simultaneously focusing on the woman's pleasure can often be very arousing to the man.

THE WISDOM OF THE PENIS

The process of erection is dependent on both physical and psychological factors. Assuming you have found that your plumbing is working and that you are getting the right amount of direct stimulation, you need to consider the possibility that the problem may be related to performance anxiety, guilt, fear, stress, or other psychological reasons. Occasional impotence, once again, may result from what Bernie Zilbergeld aptly calls "the wisdom of the penis," reminding your brain that you don't really want to be sexual at that moment. We assume that erections should be as automatic as salivation and that "real" men should be able to have sex at any moment, but neither is true. So the first thing you want to do is have a heart-to-crotch conversation and decide if you are really doing what you want to be doing. If the answer is no, tell your partner why and/or suggest a better time.

If the answer is yes, and you still have erection trouble, you may want to seek out psychological or sexual therapy. It is no wonder, given all the misinformation and hype about men's penises and male sexuality in general, that most men see sex as in some way a performance. The more you can shift your focus from how you did, how long you lasted, and how much you satisfied your partner to the pleasure that you and your partner are experiencing, the better off you and your erection will be. As Bernie Zilbergeld wisely points out, "It can help men to realize that most women are less concerned about a man's performance than they are about his reaction to it and to her. Women are more likely to get upset about the man's negative reaction to a performance problem (anger, guilt, constant apologies, withdrawal) than to the problem itself."

PHYSICAL EXHAUSTION

According to the Taoist physicians, erection trouble is caused not only by physiological or psychological problems. It can also be caused by an energetic problem—specifically, weak sexual energy. Difficulty in getting or maintaining an erection is understood as resulting from a man's physical and sexual exhaustion. Many older men who have not conserved their seed suffer from this problem. The cure for impotence is to cultivate the sexual energy while

TESTICLE MASSAGE

1. Rub your hands together to warm them up.

2. Hold one testicle between the thumb and fingers of each hand (see figure 36). (Your testicles should feel like small apricots between your fingers.)

3. Firmly but gently massage your testicles with your thumbs and fingers for a minute or two. If your testicles ache or are sensitive, rub lighter but longer, until the pain goes away. The pain is caused by a blockage, and the massage will help bring blood and sexual energy to the area, which will disperse any blockage.

4. Hold your penis up to expose your testicles and tap them with your longest finger for a minute or two (see figure 37). This helps invigorate your testes and increase sperm production.

5. Finally, hold your penis and scrotum with your thumb and forefinger (see figure 38). Now lightly pull your penis and scrotum forward with your hand as you pull back with your pelvic muscles. Then repeat, pulling to the right with your hand and to the left with your pelvic muscles. Then pull to the left with your hand and to the right with your pelvic muscles. Finish by pulling your hand down and your pelvic muscles up. Do this exercise nine, eighteen, or thirty-six times. It will keep the ducts that carry your sperm healthy.

avoiding ejaculation at all costs. As we mentioned in chapter 5, a man is generally more yang than yin. As he becomes more and more aroused, he becomes more and more yang, but after ejaculating he becomes yin. Men who have erection trouble need to become more yang and therefore must avoid ejaculation even more vigilantly than other men.

TESTICLE MASSAGE

The Taoists also developed exercises to help you generate more sexual energy. Lovemaking (using the Soft Entry technique, if necessary) and the Big Draw were a commonly prescribed duo-cultivation method. In addition, there were a number of solo-cultivation exercises that would help a man restore his sexual en-

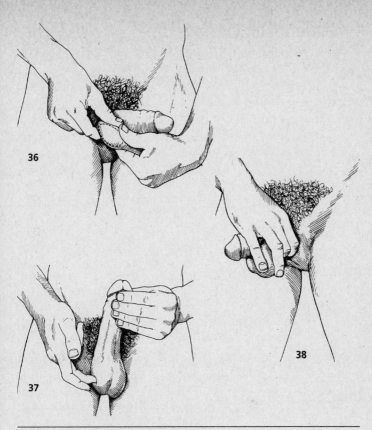

FIGURES 36–38. MASSAGING YOUR TESTICLES
TAPPING YOUR TESTICLES
STRETCHING PENIS AND TESTICLE TENDONS

ergy. According to the Taoists, your sexual energy is dependent on three things: the abundance of your sexual hormones, the strength of your kidneys, and the circulation of your bioelectric energy, or *chi*. Western medicine has confirmed that the sex hormone testosterone is produced in your testicles, and Taoists believe that you can increase the production of sex hormones by using the Testicle Massage exercise. This exercise is an excellent way to strengthen your sexual energy in general and also to relieve any pressure that you may feel after lovemaking. By massaging your testicles, you also help circulate the blood through them and keep them healthy.

A WHOLE-BODY APPROACH

The Taoists saw illness, including impotence, as an expression of the health of your whole body. They recognized that your penis was just part of the problem. Poor circulation, superficial breathing, and an unhealthy diet could all make it worse. Smoking is especially bad for your circulation, since it causes the blood vessels and arteries to constrict and interferes with your breathing. Alcohol and caffeine also drain the body and should be avoided while you are trying to strengthen your sexual energy. An erection problem is a condition that must be treated throughout your body by strengthening your sexual energy and by maintaining proper health.

Please, Sir, May I Have Some More: Enlarging Your Penis

Any man who has been in a locker room knows that there are differences in the size and shape of men's penises. But these differences have little to do with the pleasure a woman experiences during lovemaking—especially if a man practices Sexual Kung Fu. In the words of Su Nü, "There are indeed distinctions in physical endowment. Large and small, long and short, and physical differences are matters of external appearance. Deriving pleasure from sexual intercourse is a matter of inner emotion. If you first bind them with love and respect and press them with true sentiments; then of what relevance are large and small, long and short?"

Even with this and other assurances, many men still worry about the size of their penis, and quite a few men have even undergone "penile enhancement" surgery. This new surgical procedure typically involves lengthening the penis by cutting the suspensory ligament that connects the base of the penis to the pubic bone (see figure 39). In addition to the lengthening procedure, men can also have their penis "thickened" by having fat that has been liposuctioned from their thighs, pubic area, or hips injected into the shaft of the penis.[4]

IF IT AIN'T BROKE, DON'T FIX IT

What man wouldn't like a few extra inches? But before you run out and have surgery, you should know that there are serious risks.

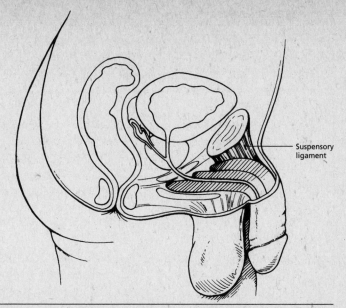

FIGURE 39.   THE SUSPENSORY LIGAMENT THAT CONNECTS THE BASE OF THE PENIS
TO THE PUBIC BONE

According to an article in the *San Francisco Chronicle,* the lengthening procedure can result in nerve damage and decreased sensation, impotence, lower angle of erection, skin protrusions, scarring,
infection, and gangrene. The thickening procedure can cause an
embolism in the heart or brain from the fat released during liposuc-
tion, tissue death from reduced blood supply in the penis caused by
too much fat in the penis, or a lumpy or lopsided penis.

The article in the *Chronicle* also describes the experience of a
thirty-five-year-old auto mechanic who had a number of complica-
tions from the surgery, including a "grotesque lump" at the base of
his penis. His penis was also black and blue for several weeks. "I
thought it was going to fall off. I thought I was left deformed for
life." He finally took his "new" penis to a urologist, who did repair
surgery. Dr. C. Eugene Carlton, president of the American Urolog-
ical Association, also states that he has heard reports of a dozen serious infections and several cases of impotence. He had to treat
one man with an infection so severe he required skin grafting to replace half the skin on his penis.

ENLARGING YOUR PENIS

1. Inhale through your nose into your throat and then swallow this bubble of air, pressing it down into your stomach. (It should not stay in your chest.)

2. Imagine this breath as a ball of energy, *chi*, which you want to push down from your stomach through your pelvis and out into your penis. This will help you bring more energy to your penis.

3. Once you have pushed this ball of energy into your penis, use the three middle fingers of your left hand to press the Million-Dollar Point between the anus and scrotum. This will lock the energy into the penis.

4. Breathe normally while keeping your fingers on the Million-Dollar Point. At the same time, begin the following stretches.

5. With the right hand, grip your penis and begin rhythmically pulling it forward and away from your body. Pull six to nine times. Then pull to the right six to nine times. Then pull to the left six to nine times. Finally, pull down six to nine times.

6. Use your thumb to rub the head of your penis. Rub the penis until it becomes erect. If your are not getting erect, pull some more while you rub, until you have an erection.

7. Holding the shaft of the penis, circle the penis at its base with your thumb and forefinger and pull forward about an inch. This forces the energy to the head of your penis. Do this nine times.

8. Pull the penis to the right with your right hand and rotate the penis in small circles. Do this six to nine times in one direction and then the other, maintaining the outward pressure. Repeat, pulling it to the left and making six to nine small circles in one direction and then the other.

9. In the final stretch, gently slap your erect penis against your inner right thigh, remembering also to keep pulling outward. Do this six to nine times and then repeat the motion against your inner left thigh.

10. After completing these stretches, soak your penis in warm water for a minute. This will help your penis absorb the warm (yang) energy and expand.

Even putting aside these medical risks and horror stories, penile-enhancement surgery is misguided according to the Tao. The *strength* of an erection is much more important than its *size*. After their suspensory ligaments have been cut, men often have a lower angle of erection and the increased fat adds girth but not strength. To have an erection your penis needs blood and sexual energy. If the penis is made too large, without enough blood and sexual energy you will have difficulty getting hard. According to Su Nü, "Long and large, but weak and soft, does not compare to short and small, but firm and hard."

IN THE LOCKER ROOM

The truth is, it is in the locker room that most men are concerned about the size of their penis—not in the bedroom. For this reason, it is worth keeping in mind that there is more variation in flaccid penises than in erect ones. Penises that look small in the locker room expand more in the bedroom than ones that look bigger in the locker room. Also, given the particular angle from which you look at your penis, it seems smaller to you than to anyone else—a cruel divine joke that is guaranteed to cause inferiority complexes. Try looking down at yourself and then look in the mirror. Surprise! You just gained an inch or two. Most men have an exaggerated sense of how big other men are, partly because of the angle of observation and partly because they don't know the facts. According to urologist Claudio Teloken, who injected 150 men with a medicine that causes erections and then measured their penises from the pubic bone to the tip of the glans, the "average" man's erect penis is 5.7 inches long. Contrary to popular belief, neither race nor body type makes any significant difference, and the size of the penis has nothing to do with sexual sensitivity.

If you are still concerned about the size of your penis, there is an ancient Taoist exercise for extending your penis that is certainly worth trying before you go to the expense and danger of surgery. It is based on exercising and stretching your penis. There is little scientific confirmation for the success of penis-enlargement exercises, but Alan and Donna Brauer report that 110 men who undertook their extensive sexual-enhancement program reported permanent increases in the size of their penis, from a quarter of an inch to an inch.[5] It is clear that lack of use can cause the penis to shrink—literally to retract into the body—so it should also stand to reason that frequent use should cause it to extend slightly.

You have no doubt noticed some shrinkage after a swim in cold water. The reason this occurs, and that some expansion may be possible, is that your penis actually extends back into your body two to four inches. These additional inches are held in place by your suspensory ligament, which is what the penile-enhancement surgeons cut. It is probable that frequent erection and sexual activity can cause this ligament to stretch, allowing the hidden part of the penis to move out of the body somewhat.

The time-tested Enlarging Your Penis exercise has been known to extend the penis by as much as an inch within a month or two, but this will depend on your body structure, your health, and your age. The exercise is more likely to work for younger men, whose bodies are still elastic. Weak circulation will make it more difficult. You can determine any gains by measuring your erect penis before you begin and over the duration of your practice. (Make sure you measure from your pubic bone to the tip of your penis and that your erection is at a ninety-degree angle from your body.) No matter what success you have in stretching your penis, this exercise also massages and energizes the entire urogenital system, including the prostate gland.

IN THE BEDROOM

If you are concerned more about the bedroom than the locker room, there is something you can do for your partner that is much better than undergoing penile surgery or even doing penis-extension exercises: Arouse her fully before entering her. If her vagina is engorged, your penis will seem larger to her. As we mentioned earlier, women generally experience the most sensation in their clitoris and the first couple of inches of their vagina, which means that even a man with a small penis can reach these most sensitive spots. The position adjustments we described in chapter 5 will also help any couple accommodate differences in genital size.

Some couples actually have the opposite problem: the man's penis is too large for his partner. Though a woman's vagina can expand considerably, this imbalance can be painful if the partners are truly mismatched. One solution is to tie a handkerchief or a shoelace around the base of the man's penis at the point of desired depth. This also has the added benefit of expanding the head of the man's penis, which can give greater pleasure to both partners. Just as you must allow your penis size to decrease about every twenty minutes to allow the blood to circulate, you must make sure to remove the handkerchief or any other tie on your penis so that the blood does not stagnate. The woman-on-top position also helps the woman control the depth and make sure intercourse does not become painful.

It is worth repeating that *if you practice Sexual Kung Fu, you and your partner's sexual desires will be so satisfied that concern about your penis size will fade into a distant memory.* You will wonder how something as insignificant as having large ears or small ears could have taken up so much mental energy. In the words of the wise and experienced Su Nü, "When two hearts are in harmony and the energy flows freely throughout the body, then the short and the small naturally become longer and larger, the soft and the weak naturally firm and hard."

How Many Sperm Does One Man Need? Raising Your Sperm Count

According to the research of Danish endocrinologist Niels Skakke-baek, sperm counts of men in the United States and twenty other countries have fallen dramatically over the last half century—by as much as 50 percent. The cause of this precipitous decline is still being debated, and possible culprits range from tight underwear to chemical pollutants. In reporting on the environmental dangers that seem at least partly to blame, University of Florida researcher Louis Guillette told a panel of U.S. Congressmen, "Every man in this room is half the man his grandfather was."[6]

Low sperm counts are a major reason that couples have difficulty conceiving a child. Given the declining sperm counts, it may not come as a surprise that infertility is an increasing problem worldwide. The World Health Organization has reported that one in ten couples is involuntarily infertile. In the United States, a staggering one in six couples is infertile—twice as many as ten years ago. It is worth mentioning that *infertility* is a vague and imprecise diagnosis that, like *impotence*, has a tendency to become stigmatized. More to the point, this diagnosis of infertility is simply made after a certain amount of time has passed (usually a year of unprotected intercourse) without conception. According to one medical textbook, "Pregnancy is the only irrefutable proof of the sperm's capability to fertilize." You are diagnosed as infertile until you conceive. Guilty until proven innocent! So even if you have a low sperm count, you may still be able to conceive a child.

Problems in ovulation are also a significant cause of infertility, and if there is no egg to fertilize, it doesn't matter how many sperm you have. Nevertheless, if there is an egg, the more sperm you have, the better the chances of your partner getting pregnant. Though only one sperm finally joins with the egg, all the sperm actually work together to get through the uterus and fallopian tubes and fertilize the egg.

If you have a low sperm count, you will be relieved to know that there are Sexual Kung Fu exercises you can use to help raise it. Engaging in nonejaculatory sex is the most important thing you can do to increase the volume, concentration, and count of your sperm. According to Western medical research, each day you do not ejaculate, you raise your sperm count by 50 to 90 million sperm.[7]

In addition to storing up your sperm, you can help your testicles produce more by shaking, massaging, and tapping them. When our testicles were able to swing freely (before tight underwear and pants), they rubbed together and against our thighs naturally, but now that we sit most of the day and spend very little time running through the jungle naked, we must help them. You can stand with pants that are loose in the crotch and shake your testicles up and down. Then rock your lumbar region and sacrum left and right and forward and back (this will help bring blood to your genital area). The Testicle Massage exercise described earlier in this chapter is also quite effective—especially step 4, which involves tapping your testicles.

My What? Preventing and Helping Prostate Problems

Many men only hear about their prostate gland when they are diagnosed with a prostate problem, such as infection, enlargement, or cancer. Almost one in ten men is eventually diagnosed with prostate cancer, which is now so common an ailment that the medical profession generally assumes that if a man lives long enough, he will develop it. According to the Taoists this disease is not inevitable, and Sexual Kung Fu can help keep your prostate healthy.

Two exercises described in chapter 3—Stopping the Stream and PC Pull-Ups—will help you to strengthen your PC muscle, which surrounds your prostate. By squeezing this muscle you can keep your prostate healthy. As we mentioned in chapter 3, the pubococcygeus is actually a group of muscles that stretch between your pubic bone ("pubo") and your coccyx ("coccygeus"). Make sure you squeeze lightly. If you squeeze too hard, you may find that you are too tense to breathe correctly. You can do the prostate exercise every day, as often as you like. Remember, as with any exercise, you may have initial soreness if you practice a lot. According to Taoism your prostate is closely related to your brain's hypothalamus, so if you squeeze correctly, you will eventually feel a sensation in your brain.

In addition to exercising your prostate, you can also massage your prostate directly, which is what the doctor does when you have a prostate infection. The doctor massages your prostate through your anus, which you can also do, as we explain in chapter 2. You can also massage your prostate by pressing in at your Million-Dollar Point and making small circles in one direction and then the other (see the Pelvic Massage exercise in chapter 3). Using the Big Draw when you self-pleasure or make love will also help keep your prostate healthy. If you have prostate problems, make sure you use the Finger Lock when you ejaculate.

One multi-orgasmic man explained his experience with prostate pain before and after he started practicing Sexual Kung Fu: "I used to have serious pain in my prostate gland that began

EXERCISE 17

HELPING YOUR PROSTATE

1. Exhale completely, at the same time lightly contracting your perineum and anus.

2. Inhale, and then as you exhale, picture your prostate, which is just above your perineum, and contract your PC muscle around your prostate.

3. Inhale and relax.

4. Repeat this exercise nine or eighteen times.

during adolescence. Several times a month, I would experience terribly sharp pain in that area that would last several minutes. One time the pain was so bad that a friend of mine claimed that my face actually turned green. Doctors suggested ejaculating regularly to relieve the pressure in the prostate gland. This helped somewhat, but I always knew that letting all that semen out was a tremendous waste of energy. When I was in my late twenties, I discovered Sexual Kung Fu. Within several weeks of practicing the PC muscle contractions, the prostate and testicle massage, and the Big Draw and Finger Lock, the problems with my prostate virtually disappeared. I have not had prostate pain for several years now, and though there was some prostate swelling initially after I stopped ejaculating, this condition gradually declined. Given the number of men who suffer from prostate trouble, these techniques are nothing short of miraculous if they work for others like they did for me."

Sex Is Not Like Pizza: Healing Sexual Trauma

There is a joke attributed to Yankees coach Yogi Berra that goes: "Sex is like pizza. When it's good, it's *really* good. And when it's bad, it's *still* pretty good." Unfortunately, sex is not really like pizza, as many men who have had negative sexual experiences can testify.

Bad sexual experiences can linger in our libidos, returning at moments of intimacy years later.

Consensual sex sometimes ends up being hurtful, but coercive sex almost always does. Over the last few years there has been an enormous increase in the reporting of sexual abuse, sexual harassment, and sexual assault. Our willingness to address these formerly taboo subjects is an extremely important societal advance. Understandably, the shocking (and not uncontested) statistics about the prevalence of these social ills have resulted in an ever-greater desire to define exactly what consensual sex is. Although most of the media attention has focused on the sexual abuse of women, men can also be victims of exploitative sex. And both women and men can experience consensual sex that goes bad.

Consent (or the lack of it) is sometimes clear and sometimes not, since sexual partners are almost never totally equal in age, strength, experience, power, and so on. In communicating sexual interest, it is best to be as explicit as possible, rather than relying on silent signals. Fortunately, as women have discovered that they are sexual beings as much as men are, we are abandoning the confusing and dangerous mixed messages of earlier generations. "No" can finally mean *No!* and "Yes" can finally mean *Yes!*

If you have experienced coercive sex or consensual sex that went bad, you may be left with sexual scars that can cause sexual or emotional problems. If this is the case, you will probably want to seek professional therapy or sex counseling. However, there are also some things you can do on your own to help you stay focused on the pleasure of the present rather than the pain of the past.

Staying present and in your body is a challenge for anyone who has experienced sexual trauma. Paying close attention to the sensations in your body, both positive and negative, is far better than allowing your thoughts to wander or to "rise above" your body, causing you to become an observer instead of a participant. The Belly Breathing and the Century Count exercises described in chapter 3 will help you improve your concentration and your ability to stay focused. Sound, whether in the form of mantras or moans, can also clear your mind of distracting thoughts. Positive

TOUCH MEDITATION

1. Sit facing one another with your legs crossed or on your heels. The lighting should be low, preferably candlelight.

2. Using both hands, start touching your body, generally from head to toe. (Avoid any parts of your body that you do not want your partner to touch and generally avoid your genitals or leave them until last.)

3. Your partner should use her hands to follow yours, touching each place that you have just touched.

4. Switch and have your partner use her hands followed by your hands to introduce you to her body.

5. Hug and feel each other breathing.

reinforcement will also help you stay present. Remind yourself as often as necessary of where you are, whom you are with, and how good it feels. When old feelings arise, it is generally best to stop what you are doing and share with your partner the feelings that are coming up.

If you do not feel comfortable discussing your sexual trauma with your partner, especially if she is a new partner, you should try to tell her what you do want now. If she is doing something that is uncomfortable or does not feel good, tell her, but do so by saying what you'd prefer her to do rather than criticizing what she is doing. If you are not feeling particularly sexual, suggest that you hold each other, massage each other, or meditate with each other by looking into one another's eyes. You can also suggest that you do the Touch Meditation exercise. It is especially good at reestablishing intimacy that has been damaged in some way.

With Touch Meditation you reconnect with your body and share with your partner the parts of your body that you feel good about sharing. You will probably find that your partner is responsive to taking it slow and developing greater intimacy before being sexual. If your mind and body are not present, you will have very little sexual energy to share with your partner. Neither you nor she will benefit much from your lovemaking, and your pleasure will be minimal. By taking it slow and stroking your entire body, you will be able to gather your sexual energy and have an experience that is both passionate and meaningful. As already mentioned, the Taoists recognized long ago that sex has great power for healing or for harm, so use this power wisely and lovingly.

CHAPTER NINE

Making Love for a Lifetime

In Taoism, our bodies are considered to be microcosms of the natural world, so we must think of ourselves and our sexuality as changing like the seasons: spring, summer, fall, winter. Yet the Taoist masters were able to turn the seasons one more time, experiencing a second springtime in old age. Consumed with the search for immortality, they found in Sexual Kung Fu a true fountain of youth. Indeed, all modern studies show that an active sex life is essential for counteracting the effects of aging and for maintaining one's health. We will now explore how sex can actually help you live longer and what specifically you need to know as your sexuality changes.

Sex and Aging

You are never too *young* to read about sex and aging. In the West, we tend to think of aging as something that happens late in life, but the aging process begins at birth, and our sexuality changes every few years. As Kinsey put it, "The sexagenarian—or octogenarian—who suddenly becomes interested in the problems of aging is nearly a lifetime beyond the point at which he became involved in that process."[1] The sooner you read this section, the better off you'll be.

You are also never too *old* to read this chapter, for according to the Tao, sex is a lifelong activity that is possible and desirable until the day you die. In the West, older men who are still interested in sex are considered lecherous—"dirty old men." The Tao never had this prejudice; on the contrary, sex was seen to be even more important for the health and longevity of men and women in old age, or what we now call *late adulthood*. The Chinese are not alone in this belief. A cross-cultural survey has shown that sex is vitally important for older men in 70 percent of cultures and for older women in 80 percent.[2]

Closer to home, a *Consumer Reports* survey demonstrated how different the realities of sexuality among the elderly are from the cultural stereotypes: among those surveyed, over 80 percent of the married men and 75 percent of the unmarried men over seventy years old remained sexually active. Fifty-eight percent had sex at least once a week, 75 percent reported "high enjoyment of sex," and 43 percent still masturbated.[3] You also shouldn't assume that your partner's sexual appetite diminishes after menopause. Many women find that their interest in sex actually increases after menopause, perhaps because of their changing hormonal levels.

In the West, we glorify adolescent male sexuality and see a man's sexual power as peaking at age eighteen and declining steadily thereafter. In the words of one sexologist, "The adolescent penis is the penis at its ultimate power. From here on until the end of life, there is a gradual tapering off." The problem comes from a general misunderstanding of sexual power in the West. In terms of potency, it is true that a man's ability to produce sperm peaks during early adulthood, but this is important only if we are concerned with reproduction. A woman's fertility and ability to bear a child also peak in early adulthood.

However, in terms of pleasure rather than potency, a man's ability to satisfy his partner and himself only increases as he gains more experience and control. Although a man may no longer get hard instantly or be able to shoot his ejaculate as far as he could as an adolescent, these changes hardly compromise his ability as a lover. The Taoists knew that as a man leaves the fever of adolescent sexuality with its quick ejaculation, his Sexual Kung Fu practice and his partner's pleasure only increase.

AS YOUR BODY CHANGES

Inevitably, there are a number of physiological changes that take place as you age. For example, if you are over fifty, you probably need more direct stimulation of your genitals to get an erection than you did when you were younger: this is not because your sexual appetite or your attraction to your partner has disappeared, but simply because your physiology changes as you get older. Also, your erection is probably less firm and angles down more than it did when you were younger. In addition, if you ejaculate, the force of the ejaculate is less and your recovery time is longer.

These changes of decreased physical strength and stamina are no different from changes in any other physical ability as you get older. You don't expect to be able to run as fast or as far at sixty as you could at twenty. But there is one difference between sex and sports with regard to aging: your ability in bed may actually improve. Older men can actually maintain an erection longer than before (although if you lose your erection for whatever reason, it will be more difficult to regain). This will make it easier for you to satisfy your partner and to become multi-orgasmic without ejaculating. In Dunn and Trost's recent study, half the men had become multi-orgasmic after the age of thirty-five. A number had become multi-orgasmic between the ages of forty-five and fifty-five. And the older men who had learned to become multi-orgasmic, all now over fifty, were still multi-orgasmic and going strong.[4]

Most of the Western sexual literature also suggests that the intensity of the sexual experience diminishes as a man ages. This is not the case according to the Tao. The Taoists do not measure intensity according to the number of genital contractions, which do decrease as you get older. Since they recognize that sexual energy is a whole-body affair, they judge the intensity of sex on a man's ability to cultivate and circulate his sexual energy, which only increases as he gets more experience. Your sexuality will no doubt change over time, and you may miss some of the feeding frenzy of youth, but the more refined pleasures of older age are just as delectable, if not more so.

YOUR BODY AND SEX

We hope you now understand that sexuality for the older man is not a slippery slope to sexual inadequacy. Still, you will find that you are able to climb much more easily to the peaks of pleasure if you observe the basic needs of your older body. First, a healthy body and regular exercise are essential. One reason so many people's sex lives shrivel as they age is that their bodies become weak or ill. The wisdom of the East and all physiological studies in the West have concluded that exercise not only improves sexual ability but increases sexual desire and orgasms. Your abdomen, hips, buttocks, and thighs are especially important large muscles, as is the smaller PC muscle we discussed earlier. Keeping these muscles strong is essential for maintaining sexual vitality. Although swimming, jogging, and other Western sports are excellent ways of maintaining physical health (as long as they are not overdone), regular sex is as important, if not more so. *Use it or lose it* quite accurately describes the aging male body.

According to the Tao, a great deal of sexual energy leaks out of our anus and buttocks. Try squeezing your buttocks together and you will see how powerful this muscle is for containing energy and sending it up your spine. The Taoist doctors considered the strength of a person's anal sphincter an important sign of health. A loose, weak sphincter is a sign of poor health; a tight, strong sphincter, a sign of good health. You can strengthen your anus and buttocks by using the following exercise. In addition, this exercise will help you relieve stress while energizing your body and developing your sexual control. It also will help energize your prostate and Cowper's glands and circulate your blood and strengthen your erections. It has even been known to help cure hemorrhoids.

EXERCISE 19

STRENGTHENING YOUR ANUS

1. Exhale completely through your nose and then pump and pull up the muscles in your anus and buttocks for several seconds. (You will be repeatedly squeezing and releasing these muscles.)

2. Inhale slowly and relax.

3. Repeat steps 1 and 2 nine, eighteen, or thirty-six times, or until your groin and anus start to feel warm. This energy may gradually spread to your head and down to your navel, or you can draw it up consciously to the tailbone and the sacrum, and up the spine to the head along the Microcosmic Orbit. Rest and spiral the energy in the head eighteen to thirty-six times. If you feel too much energy, remember to touch your tongue to the roof of your mouth to let the energy come down to your navel (see chapter 3).

EJACULATION AND AGING

By now it should be obvious that the place you lose the most energy is out your penis through ejaculating. For aging men, as we discussed in chapter 3, nonejaculatory lovemaking is even more important as each ejaculation becomes more exhausting to the body. As we mentioned once before, the long-lived Chinese physician Sun Ssu-miao recommended that men at forty ejaculate no more than once in ten days, that men of fifty ejaculate no more than once in twenty days, and that men at sixty no longer ejaculate. These are maximum amounts, and if you are able to transform your sexual energy by drawing it up, the less frequently you ejaculate, the better off you will be. This may be difficult at first if you are just starting to practice Sexual Kung Fu, but once you experience the pleasure of nonejaculatory orgasms and understand their health benefits, you will be extremely motivated to learn quickly. Even better, if you start when you are younger, your appetite for ejaculation will quickly decrease and as you get older you will have little or no interest in it.

Sun Ssu-miao's recommended frequencies are just guidelines, and every few years you can simply decrease the number of times you ejaculate. This will naturally allow you to keep your frequency of ejaculation in line with your increasing needs for conservation. It is interesting to point out that even Masters and Johnson recognized that men do not need to ejaculate every time they make love, especially once they reach the age of fifty. If a man recognizes this important point, they concluded, "he is potentially a most effective sexual partner."[5] Once again, it is important that you not become obsessed with nonejaculation and that you not berate yourself if you do ejaculate. If you ejaculate, let go and enjoy it.

Keeping Love Alive

In the West, we tend to think that love and passion peak on the wedding night and die shortly thereafter.[6] The reasons for this decline are never fully explained to us, but it seems that after the thrill of courtship is over, boredom (supposedly) sets in. For Taoists, the wedding night is just the beginning of a lifetime of expanding love and intimacy. With Sexual Kung Fu, love and sex are better at fifty or even sixty than they are at twenty. Here's why.

MAINTAINING THE SEXUAL CHARGE

According to Taoism, our attraction to our partner is dependent on the strength of the yin-yang charge that exists between us. The greater the charge, the greater the passion. The lesser the charge, the lesser the passion. The loss of this charge is the reason many relationships become flat or boring. (It is also the reason many of these couples experience a flicker of passion after one of the partners has been away on a business trip, since temporary separation tends to recharge the polarity of the partners.)

One of the main reasons for the loss of this charge over time is ejaculatory sex. When the man ejaculates, he depletes his yang charge. Whether consciously or not, the man also starts to realize he is being exhausted by lovemaking. This can often lead to resentment and a desire to withhold sex. Although as mentioned the more common stereotype is of the ever-desirous husband and the frigid wife, the truth is that men as often as women determine the frequency of lovemaking. Over time, the depletion of a man's energy and specifically his yang charge can lead to disinterest and boredom for both partners.

Some couples are able to temporarily recharge their relationship by sleeping in separate beds or spending time apart. Duo cultivation (described in chapter 5) allows couples to maintain this polarity and keep their relationship fully charged. There is no reason that love must go flat or that boredom must set in. Though there are numerous reasons that people have extramarital affairs, boredom and sexual dissatisfaction are certainly two of the main ones. Maintaining the power of attraction in your relationship decreases the desire to seek out the charge of a new lover. Inexhaustible pleasure exists in every couple if they are able to conserve and exchange sexual energy. One multi-orgasmic man describes his and his partner's experience: "The practice has deepened our relationship, our love is growing, and the magnetic attraction for each other seems not to decrease, but rather to intensify."

Contrary to the stereotypical idea that sex in marriage is unsatisfying, most studies show that married couples have *better* sex with one another than they have in affairs. Bernie Zilbergeld points out that men and women tend to have *less* variety and to experiment *less* in affairs than in marriage and that women tend to be far more orgasmic with their husbands than with lovers.[7] Women are not the only ones who are more orgasmic with their spouses. Kinsey also found that men often fail to reach orgasm in extramarital affairs but almost never experience this failure with their wives.[8]

Good sex is not the only benefit of long-term relationships. A study conducted at the University of California at Berkeley concluded that couples in long-term marriages become happier and more affectionate as they age. In our society, we endlessly praise new love in songs, literature, and films. We dismiss love between older couples as passionless and boring. "What we actually thought we would see is a kind of fatigue quality in these relationships," said Robert Levenson, one of the researchers. "But that's not what we see. They're vibrant, they're alive, they're emotional, they're fun, they're sexy, they're not burned out." Recent biological studies suggest that the presence of a long-term lover increases the body's production of endorphins, natural painkillers that give partners a sense of serenity and security in their lives.[9]

Couples who choose to love one another without getting married can have lovemaking that is just as holy and intimate as the lovemaking of those who have the state's official stamp of approval—as long as they practice the union of yin and yang. Yet it is important to keep in mind that it takes years to reach the heights of physical, emotional, and spiritual intimacy and to master the union of yin and yang. It is said in Taoism that it takes seven years to know a woman's body, seven years to know her mind, and seven years to know her spirit. The saying does not mean that after this you stop learning or start growing bored; rather, it simply means that it takes twenty-one years to really get acquainted.

The Seasons of Our Sex Lives

Relationships, the Taoists knew, are not linear. They do not peak on the wedding night or on any other night. Rather, they wax and wane with the cycles of family, work, health, and even nature. It is important to be aware of these cycles and to know how to live harmoniously with them, in and out of the bedroom.

First and foremost is the need to communicate with your partner about these cycles, to be aware of your own waxing and waning desire, and to be able to talk about it in such a way that neither of you feels judged or blamed. Many women (and an increasing number of men) see a direct correlation between their partner's desire and their own attractiveness. It is important for you and your partner to escape this trap by recognizing that sex has as much to do with your hearts, minds, and spirits as it does with your bodies.

Western materialism encourages us to look at one another's bodies as commodities. We are taught to "get off" on a woman's full breasts or a man's washboard stomach. Our fetishes and media-generated fantasies are endless. So when our bodies age, we think we should stop having sex or should look for partners who are "new and improved." Taoists view the body as dynamic, realizing that the real charge comes from the interplay of subtle energies and not from the pounding together of two hard, static bodies.

Joseph Kramer explains the difference in Taoist sexuality: "In the Eastern tradition, there is eye contact almost all the time during sex. 'I am having sex with *you*. I am breathing with *you*. I am relaxed with *you*. I am connected in the heart with *you*. I am connected in the genitals with *you*.' Sex in a Taoist relationship is better at sixty than at twenty." Legs, stomachs, and genitals get old, but eyes just grow wiser.

SEX BEGINS LONG BEFORE YOU TOUCH

Since sex is a dynamic force, you need to be very conscious of the energy you bring to it. Sex really begins as much as forty-eight hours before you actually make love; the energy and emotions that you have accumulated during this time follow you into the bedroom. So, a day or two before making love, try to work through any negative emotions, especially anger, that will block the exchange of energy between you. The more calm and connected you are when you begin, the easier it will be to reach higher levels of intimacy and ecstasy. Clearly, few couples plan sex two days in advance, so you need to be conscious of your emotions in general and try to work them through as soon as possible.

Foreplay, too, begins before you touch one another. The setting you create—candles, soothing music, and romantic, loving words—will help harmonize your energies. During and after lovemaking be sure to stay present with your partner: remember the eyes. You are trying to experience a more profound state of being together, not just a momentary climax.

If lovemaking becomes routine or mechanical, stop for a while. This will allow the polar passion between you to recharge. Yet don't forget the importance of touch and intimacy. The fact that you are not making love does not mean you should not hold each other or be emotionally intimate. In fact, observing a "sex fast" can allow you to focus on these other parts of your relationship, which are as important. Focus on the quality of your love, and the quality of your sex will naturally improve.

THE CYCLES OF YOUR DESIRE

You will also find that the cycles of your sexual desire do not always coincide. At times you will feel more desire than your partner, and at times you will feel less. No one who is truly in touch with his or her body and emotions wants sex all the time. However, what should you do if one of you is interested in sex but the other one is not? There are several options that correspond to different ways of making love.

Let's assume that tonight you are feeling aroused and your partner is not. Of course, if your partner is interested, she can pleasure you orally or manually. If she is not in the mood, she may be willing to touch or hold you as you pleasure yourself. If she is not in the mood for this, either, she may be willing to exchange nonsexual touch. You can exchange a great deal of powerful, healing energy through holding each other or touching each other. (The Touch Meditation exercise described in chapter 8 is one option.)

If sex is specifically what you need and sex is specifically not what your partner is interested in, you can of course make love to yourself (that is, self-pleasure). Remember, all of us have yin and yang, feminine and masculine aspects, within ourselves. Self-intercourse, or the union of these two aspects, is a very powerful part of the Taoist practice. Michael Winn explains: "It is possible to harness the sexual energy of the genitals and kidneys and the emotional energy of the heart through meditation. This meditation practice, known as the water-and-fire method (called the *Lesser Kan* and *Li*), allows you to literally make love inside yourself and have an even higher level of orgasm, one that dissolves the boundaries between your body and spirit. This practice also has a great many health benefits and was traditionally referred to as a method of repairing the body and the soul."

Because of the societal stigma regarding masturbation, many people are too embarrassed to self-pleasure when anyone else, including their partner, is around. However, if this natural part of human sexuality can be discussed in an open sexual dialogue, you will find that you can harmonize your individual sexual cycles with ease and a great deal of pleasure.

INTEGRATING YOUR SEXUAL ENERGY INTO YOUR LIFE

Often people turn to sex when all they really need is loving touch. As one multi-orgasmic man explains, "The biggest discovery for me was that I could have sex with my clothes on, just by being with somebody and sharing the energy. It feels very sexual, just touching and holding hands and feeling the sexual energy flow through your bodies. This is really sexual freedom, because sex is not just something you engage in periodically. Your sexuality is integrated into your whole life, adding color and intensity, interest and passion to everything."

If you are a parent dealing with the demands of work and family or a person who has an extremely demanding career, the increased energy that comes from practicing Sexual Kung Fu can help you avoid burning out. The ever-increasing demands of work and family in our overcommitted, overworked, overstressed lives are enough to exhaust anyone. Once you are able to cultivate your energy both in and out of the bedroom, you will find that you have more energy than you ever thought possible.

FANTASIES

Many Western sex experts recommend having an active fantasy life, and indeed fantasies can help you to generate sexual energy when you are self-pleasuring. When you are with your partner, however, there is a danger in relying on sexual fantasies. The exchange of yin and yang energy with your partner is real, not imaginary. If you focus your sexual attention on some idealized lover or some pornographic image, you will not be able to feel the real and profound flow of energy between you and your partner. Fantasies prevent you from being present and from appreciating what is truly fantastic about your partner and about your potential to experience the heights of ecstasy together.

NATURAL RHYTHMS

Finally, remember to observe the general rhythms of your body and of nature. Avoid making love right after a big meal. After you have eaten, your body needs to focus its blood and energy on digestion. When you finish a meal, you should be satisfied, not stuffed, with a little hunger remaining. (As the food settles, you will become full.) When you finish lovemaking, you also should be satisfied but not sated, with a little desire left over. (As your energy settles, you will become content.)

If you are ill, remember to make love with your partner on top so that you can absorb her healing energy. And remember the seasons of nature. Plants and animals all reproduce in the spring. Though humans are unique in their ability to make love all year long, don't expect yourself or your partner to be as sexually active in the fall and winter as you are in the spring and summer.

Sexual Kung Fu offers you the potential for multi-orgasmic lovemaking far beyond what most people settle for in their sex lives, but this does not mean that you need to reach the heights of ecstasy every time you are intimate with your partner. Listen to the rhythms of your body and your desire.

AVOID INCREASING THE STAKES

Every time a sexual possibility is introduced to Western readers, the sexual stakes tend to get raised. Once women's orgasms were "discovered," couples were expected to start having simultaneous orgasms. When some women were found to be multi-orgasmic and to have G spots, all women were expected to have multiple orgasms and G spots. Every man has the potential to become multi-orgasmic and to experience whole-body orgasms, but not every man will want to experience them every time. Try to avoid creating performance expectations and anxiety. The Taoist sexual techniques we are teaching are also called the *healing love*. If you focus on love and healing, for yourself and for your partner, the rest will naturally follow.

No Free Love

Monogamy is back, even if as nothing more than a health precaution. But monogamy is much more than an onerous requirement of the times. With the right partner, it can be a crucible for a most powerful alchemical process of physical pleasure, emotional intimacy, and spiritual growth.

If the indiscriminate accumulation of sexual energy were the goal of Sexual Kung Fu, it might be best to sleep with as many people as possible and to exchange energy with all of them. And indeed, there were ancient texts that recommended this practice. But it is not just the amount of sexual energy you have that is important, it is also the quality of that energy. The goal of Sexual Kung Fu is to eventually transform sexual energy into more refined and subtle energies of the heart, mind, and spirit.

SEXUAL ENERGY AND EMOTIONS

If you are sleeping with people who have a great many negative emotions (such as anger or sadness), you will internalize their emotions. *No matter how much latex you put between you and your partner, you are always exchanging emotional and spiritual (as well as sexual) energy.* So avoid violating your bodily, emotional, and spiritual integrity by having sex with someone you do not respect and love. In choosing a partner, you are quite literally choosing your spiritual destiny.

In reality, men (and women) who have not found a loving partner have sexual urges that need satisfaction—an itch that needs to be scratched. If this is your situation, you would be better off practicing solo cultivation and learning to circulate and transform your sexual energy. This training period will allow you to raise the level of your internal energy; eventually you will attract an equally aware and mature partner. If you sleep with someone you do not love, your energy will be in disharmony and either drain you or cause imbalances. For the same reason, you should make love with your partner only when you feel true affection for her. If you feel you must sleep with women you do not love, try to be as kind and loving to them as you can be. Otherwise, it will be impossible for you to truly practice Sexual Kung Fu.

Quite a few men find they are attracted to or interested in being in a relationship with more than one woman. Few men, however, can love more than one woman at a time and feel true serenity. If you think you can, be prepared to spend a great deal of effort trying to transform and balance their energies.

Remember, sexual energy simply magnifies whatever emotions you are feeling. Sex is the most powerful tool for cultivating a relationship and joining our lives together, but it can also be a sharp weapon that can sever those ties and leave lasting scars. As many who experienced the sexual revolution of the 1960s learned, there is no "free love": sexual knowledge comes at a high price and should be cherished accordingly.

Teaching Our Sons

Chances are you were not told about Sexual Kung Fu when you were growing up and learning about your sexuality. Few people are so fortunate. Most boys learn very little about sexuality and practically nothing that is of use. They are left to grope in the dark for sexual intimacy and pleasure. As one multi-orgasmic man explained, "For me, discovering Taoist sexuality was like coming across information and guidance that I felt should have been explained to me from the beginning. It felt like the right way to make love, and the old way seemed so ridiculous, embarrassing, even selfish." You have a chance to help your son avoid this situation and save him from a great deal of the fear and frustration we mistakenly assume is an inevitable part of growing up.

NO BIRDS AND NO BEES

Both parents have an important role to play in the sexual education of their sons and daughters, but since this is primarily a book for men, we will focus specifically on fathers and sons, although much of what we have to say is applicable to mothers and daughters as well. When most people think about discussions of sex between fathers and sons, they generally think of the famous man-to-man talks about the birds and the bees when a boy comes of age. Kids grow up much too fast today to make quaint discussions about birds and bees of any use—if they ever were. Adolescence is in reality much too late a time in your son's development for you to begin establishing a dialogue with him about sexuality.

If you succeed in maintaining an open relationship with your son, such a talk will never be necessary. Children's curiosity about sex begins early, and their sexuality begins even earlier. Anyone who has witnessed an infant boy touching and pulling on his penis and scrotum (often quite hard!) knows that this is not just random exploration. The boy is receiving pleasure—more than he receives when, for example, he pulls on his toes.

Babies are sexual beings, or perhaps we should say *sensual* beings, since we generally associate sexuality with later stages of development. However, their physical and genital pleasure is undeniable—as much as we try to deny it. Freud called infant sensuality "polymorphous perversity," but there is nothing perverse about it except our own attempts to repress it. How you respond to your son's explorations of and questions about his and your bodies will teach him a great deal about his sexuality. *Developing a healthy, loving relationship to your sexuality and encouraging him to develop the same with his sexuality is the first thing you can do for your son.*

YOUR RELATIONSHIP TO YOUR PARTNER

Children also learn a great deal about intimacy from watching their parents. How you treat your wife or partner will be a model for how your son should treat girls and, later, women. Learning about sex is really learning about sex roles, about communication, about love. What you model will have a much greater impact on your son than what you say, so remember that you are always teaching—when you are hollering at one another as well as when you are holding hands.

In this culture, we worry about children seeing their parents being physically affectionate with one another, but there is nothing wrong with children witnessing these expressions of love. In fact, there may be a problem with them not witnessing it. Its absence not only leaves children often wondering whether their parents love each other but also leaves them without models of how to express affection to their own partners. *Modeling a healthy, loving relationship with your partner is the second thing you can do for your son—not to mention for your partner and yourself.*

YOUR RELATIONSHIP TO YOUR SON

Many men are becoming more involved in child care than their fathers were, and this naturally leads to more affectionate and loving father-son relationships. However, a lot of fathers still feel uncomfortable expressing affection, especially physical affection, toward their sons—holding them, hugging them, or kissing them.

Or, if they are able to do this with their young sons, they quickly stop as the boys grow older. Many of these men never experienced this love from their fathers and have no model for how to express it.

Some men worry that if they are too affectionate, their boys will become soft, or sissies, or gay. There is no evidence in support of any of these ideas, but it is clear that homophobia in our culture prevents men from expressing their affection for one another and, most tragically, for their sons. Over the last ten years, another issue has begun to prevent fathers from being physically affectionate toward their sons or daughters. The legitimate concern over protecting children from sexual abuse and incest has led to a suspicion of all male physical affection—since most of the perpetrators, although certainly not all, are men.

Touch is the most basic of human needs, and several studies report that babies who did not receive enough of it died. But babies are not the only ones who need touch. Your son will need your loving touch throughout his life. Don't be surprised, however, if your son goes through stages in which he refuses your affection—especially around adolescence, when he may be concerned about his peers' opinions or may be trying to become more independent. However, if you have maintained an open and loving relationship with him, this separation will be only temporary. Martial artist and actor Chuck Norris recounted one of his greatest joys in raising his two sons: "One of my biggest gratifications today is that my grown-up sons aren't embarrassed to kiss me hello or good-bye in front of anyone and that they come willingly to me for advice or help if they have problems."

Physical affection is just part of a loving relationship. Emotional intimacy and respect for your son are essential for keeping an open dialogue. Norris, whose father was alcoholic, explains how he tried to present a different role model: "I wanted my sons to know that I was there, that I cared, and that I was always in their corner. I am very close to my sons. I have played with them, listened to their problems, held them in my arms when they were hurt, and shared most of the major events, crises, and successes of their lives."[10] Listening to your son and acknowledging his feelings and his fears will allow him to know he can come to you. If you are willing to hear his pain, he will also be able to share with you his questions about pleasure. *Building a healthy, loving relationship with your son is no doubt the most important thing you can do for him.*

SHARING TAOIST SEXUALITY WITH OUR SONS

Though people are never too old to benefit from the Tao, the earlier they begin to practice, the more they will gain. This is also true for our sons. If you are able to share with your son some of the Taoist insights in this book, you will help him avoid a great deal of suffering and wasted energy.

Since sexual practices are done in privacy, your son cannot learn from your actions. Sexual Kung Fu is something you must tell him about through words—your own or others'.

Long before boys are interested in sex, they experience sexual energy. Boys (and men) get erections and aroused for all sorts of reasons—boredom, among others. (Remember those "woodies" during math class?) One multi-orgasmic man described his experience: "My son called to me from the bathroom one morning and said, 'Dad, I can't pee.' I went into the bathroom and noticed that he had woken up with an erection, which was preventing him from being able to pee. I taught him the Cool Draw, which he has been able to use ever since to manage his sexual energy." Boys are often tortured by their inability to understand and control their sexual energy. If you can help your son understand how to channel this vital energy, you will save him from an enormous amount of sexual frustration.

Young people, however, are often not able to understand the Tao. In the words of Dr. Sun Ssu-miao in his *Priceless Prescriptions*, "When a man is in his youth, he usually does not understand the Tao. Or even if he does hear or read about it, he is not likely to believe it fully and practice it. When he reaches his vulnerable old age, he will, however, realize the significance of the Tao. But by then it is often too late, for he is usually too sick to benefit fully from it."

You can wait for an opportunity when your son has approached you for advice, or you can give him this book or other materials to read, explaining that you wish you had read about these practices when you were his age. If you leave this book on your bookshelf or out in a conspicuous place, you may find that he reads it on his own, but it is important for him to realize that he does not have to lock himself in his bedroom or the bathroom to read it. You may worry that he should not read books (such as this one) that are explicit about sexuality until he reaches an appropriate age, but the appropriate age is really when he is curious enough to want to read them. Rest assured that he will not read them before he is ready, and that when he is ready, he will learn about sex one way or another.

Sexuality, Secrecy, and the Tao

It should be quite clear by now that Taoism, unlike many other spiritual traditions, encourages us to acknowledge the fact that we are embodied and that sexuality is a vital part of our humanity. For most Westerners who have been taught to be ashamed of their bodies in one way or another, this is a revolutionary idea. Ironically (some would say hypocritically), Western culture titillates at the same time that it condemns. So, for most people who are used to seeing sex being used to sell everything from beer to automobiles, the idea that sexuality is also a spiritual practice is equally revolutionary.

In this book, we have tried to explain the ancient Taoist insights about love and lovemaking and how they can be used by people today. If you do nothing more than practice the techniques in this book, your life will certainly be enriched. However, we would be negligent if we did not explain that sexuality is just part of the Taoist practice and that there are equally powerful insights and exercises for cultivating your body, your emotions, your mind, and your spirit outside the bedroom as well.

The medical traditions of Taoism, known in the West as Chinese medicine and acupuncture, have helped countless people regain their health; *chi-kung* and Tai-chi exercises have been the foundation of the internal martial arts now popular around the world; and the core philosophical text of Taoism, the *Tao Te Ching* (pronounced *DOW DE JING*), is one of the most translated and read works of world literature. In addition, over the last twenty years, the arts of the bedchamber have begun to transform the sexual lives of people all over the globe. Taoism has a great deal of practical wisdom to offer—wisdom that can help people of any religion live healthy and meaningful lives today.

As we mentioned in the introduction, Mantak Chia and his wife, Maneewan, developed the Healing Tao, and they have written numerous books explaining the various parts of this health system. There are over three hundred Healing Tao instructors in cities around the world who can help you in your practice. If you are interested in exploring other aspects of the practice, you should read other Healing Tao books or contact an instructor (see the appendix). If you and your partner are interested specifically in reading more about the sexual practices, you can read Mantak Chia's two more-advanced books, *Taoist Secrets of Love: Cultivating Male Sexual Energy* (written with Michael Winn) and *Healing Love Through the Tao: Cultivating Female Sexual Energy* (written with Maneewan Chia). There are also many excellent books about and teachers of Taoist practices that are not connected with the Healing Tao. Taoism does not seek converts, so it has been less visible than some of the other major spiritual traditions, but if you look for teachers, you will find them.

The philosophy and practices that we have taught in this book were for millennia closely guarded secrets handed down from master to disciple after years of training. We have presented them here because we believe that human culture as a whole can benefit from their dissemination. Carnal confusion is just one of the many dilemmas we face today, but as we heal ourselves and our relationships, we will begin to heal the planet itself—for, according to the Tao, we are as much a part of nature as nature is a part of us.[11] We believe that this healing must begin in the bedroom, for it is here that the next generation is conceived. It is through love and sex that humanity continues, and it is in loving and in making love that the power of transformation is perhaps greatest.

However, these teachings are not to be taken any less seriously or valued any less because you did not have to pay a million gold pieces or study for a decade with a master to learn them. Cherish them and they will reward you in manifold ways. Read, reread, practice, and share them with others. The more pleasure you give, the more pleasure you receive. The more you heal, the more you are healed. This is the true secret of Taoist sexuality.

INTRODUCTION

1. After reading these accounts, Herant Katchadourian, M.D., author of the standard textbook *Fundamentals of Human Sexuality*, concluded: "The ancient Chinese clearly understood the distinction between ejaculatory and non-ejaculatory orgasm. Those who mastered the art of achieving the latter obviated the refractory period [in other words, didn't lose their erection], which made it possible for them to engage in prolonged coitus with multiple nonejaculatory orgasms" (p. 292).

2. In conducting his famous studies of male sexuality, Kinsey discovered that "orgasm may occur without the emission of semen. . . . These males experience real orgasm which they have no difficulty in recognizing, even if it is without ejaculation." See Kinsey et al., *Sexual Behavior in the Human Male*, pp. 158–59.

3. Hartman and Fithian, *Any Man Can*, p. 157.

4. Natalie Angier, *New York Times*, Dec. 3, 1992, front page.

CHAPTER ONE: THE PROOF IS IN YOUR PANTS

1. Many of the people who have denied that men can be multi-orgasmic have confused orgasm and ejaculation. Pioneering sex researchers William Masters and Virginia Johnson titled one chapter in their 1966 book, *Human Sexual Response*, "The Male Orgasm (Ejaculation)." In their research they found that only a few of their subjects seemed capable of repeated orgasm *after they had ejaculated*. Katchadourian, however, explains: "More recent evidence suggests that multiple orgasm is not that rare if a man experiences orgasm without ejaculation." Even Masters and Johnson eventually distinguished between orgasm as "sudden, rhythmic muscular contractions in the pelvic region and elsewhere in the body that release accumulated sexual tension and the mental sensations accompanying that experience" and ejaculation as simply "the release of semen." Taoist sexuality has always taught men to have multiple orgasms, not multiple ejaculations.

2. The Reichian school of psychotherapy makes a distinction between *climax*, as the muscular contractions in the genitals, and *orgasm*, which it defines as contractions that spread throughout the entire body. Although this distinction will prove useful in learning to separate climax (and orgasm) from ejaculation, it also seems too rigid. On the continuum of sexual pleasure, the line between climax and orgasm is often blurry. So, for the purposes of this book, we will talk about climax (or genital contractions) as one aspect of orgasm.

3. Dunn and Trost, "Male Multiple Orgasms: A Descriptive Study," *Archives of Sexual Behavior*, p. 382.

4. The findings were published in the journal *Nature*. Voorhies writes, "Sex and death are two fundamental but poorly understood aspects of life. They

are often thought to be linked because reproduction requires the diversion of limited resources from somatic [bodily] growth and maintenance. This diversion of resources in mated animals, often called a cost of reproduction, is usually expressed as a reduction in life span in mated animals. . . . The reduction of mated male life span seems to be caused by additional sperm production and not by the physical activity of mating. This conclusion is supported by observations that a mutation reducing sperm production increased mean life span by about 65% in both mated males and hermaphrodites. . . . This contradicts the traditional biological assumption that large [eggs] are much costlier to produce than small sperm." Wayne A. Van Voorhies, "Production of Sperm Reduces Nematode Lifespan," *Nature* 360 (3 December 1992): 456–58.

CHAPTER TWO: KNOW THYSELF

1. Western medicine has identified: (1) a latent (filling) phase; (2) a tumescent (swelling) stage; (3) a full-erection stage; and (4) a rigid-erection stage. Pre- and posterection stages (flaccid and detumescent, respectively) are also sometimes added.

2. Several recent studies have raised the concern that vasectomy may be linked to prostate cancer. The jury is still out, but Dr. Stuart S. Howards writes in the *Western Journal of Medicine,* "The possible relationship between vasectomy and prostate cancer has to be viewed with some skepticism because two other studies, one which had long-term follow-up, did not find any effect. In addition, there is no biologically plausible explanation for a relationship between vasectomy and prostate cancer" (vol. 160, no. 2 [February 1994]: 166). Since doctors do not know what causes prostate cancer, it is very difficult for Western medicine to explain any connection between it and vasectomy.

3. Many observers and skeptics of Eastern sexuality have wrongly confused retrograde ejaculation with the nonejaculation prescribed by the Taoists.

CHAPTER THREE: BECOMING A MULTI-ORGASMIC MAN

1. Genesis 38: 8–10. According to biblical law, when a man died without any children it was his brother's responsibility to impregnate the dead man's wife in order to carry on his brother's line.

2. In the West, medicine and morality have, unfortunately, often been linked. Beginning in 1758 with the publication of *Onania, or a Treatise upon the Disorders Produced by Masturbation* by Swiss physician S. A. Tissot, Western medicine and especially psychiatry have made unsubstantiated claims that masturbation causes insanity. Most of the argument was based on the observation that mental patients masturbate. No one bothered to ask whether masturbation might be a natural part of (uninhibited) human sexuality and whether the sane and insane might both masturbate, just as they both eat and sleep. (According to the Tao, excessive ejaculation in both the sane and the insane can lead to a "brain drain.") In his 1882 book *Psychopathia Sexualis,* Richard von Krafft-Ebing, one of the world's leading psychiatrists at the time, went so far as to say that all nonreproductive sex was abnormal and sick.

3. Kinsey found that 95 percent of American men who had a high school education had masturbated by the time they were twenty-one. The percentage among college grads was even higher.

4. M. Hunt, *Sexual Behavior in the 1970s,* and R. Levin and A. Levin, "Sexual Pleasure," *Redbook* (Sept. 1975), 51–58, quoted in Zilbergeld, *The New Male Sexuality,* p. 128.

5. The researchers concluded, "masturbation is like using erotica and having frequent thoughts of sex—not an outlet so much as a component of a sexually active lifestyle." See Michael et al., *Sex in America,* pp. 158–165.

6. With modern technology, we are now able to observe the increasing activity of the sperm that occurs with sexual arousal. From relative immotility, your sperm begin whipping their tails at a phenomenal speed. This mechanical energy is one of the obvious sources of sexual energy for men.

CHAPTER FOUR: KNOW YOUR PARTNER

1. Anthony Pietropinto and Jacqueline Simenaut, *Beyond the Male Myth* (New York: Signet, 1977), quoted in Brauer and Brauer, *The ESO Ecstasy Program,* p. 27.

2. Barbach, *For Each Other,* p. 66. See also Belzer, Whipple, and Moger, "On Female Ejaculation."

3. Sigmund Freud, the founder of modern psychology and generally a brilliant theoretician, really got this one wrong. In 1920, he argued that the clitoris was an inferior version of the penis and that women therefore had what he called "penis envy." He concluded that women who were clitorally orgasmic were sexually immature and that "real women" had vaginal orgasms. Pretty loopy, huh? Unfortunately, it wasn't until 1953 that Kinsey rescued clitoral orgasms from the stigma of immaturity by demonstrating that half of the women he interviewed had orgasms through stimulation of their clitoris and that there was no evidence that they were any less mature than women who had orgasms through stimulation of their vaginas.

CHAPTER FIVE: BECOMING A MULTI-ORGASMIC COUPLE

1. Clearly there were power relations in Chinese bedrooms, and the whole institution of polygamy, multiple wives, and concubines among the nobility was fraught with power dynamics. In addition, many of the later Taoist texts describe a battle of the sexes in bed, but the earliest texts were clearly more concerned with pleasure (especially the woman's) and health for both partners.

2. *I Ching* 1.5.

3. "The rate of infection for people outside of present highest risk groups and their sexual partners is estimated to be about 1/100,000," Institute for Advanced Study of Human Sexuality, *Complete Guide to Safer Sex,* p. 43.

CHAPTER SIX: SATISFACTION GUARANTEED

1. Hartman and Fithian, p. 157.

2. In the 1950s, sex researcher Alfred Kinsey reported that three-quarters of all men were ejaculating within two minutes after beginning intercourse.

Most women require substantially longer than two minutes to experience an orgasm, let alone multiple orgasms. Twenty-five years later, the *Redbook Report of Female Sexuality* reported that three-quarters of the women interviewed were regularly orgasmic during intercourse and that most of these women needed at least six to ten minutes of thrusting (Tavris and Sadd, *The Redbook Report on Female Sexuality,* New York: Delacorte Press, 1977). According to a recent national sex survey sponsored by the University of Chicago, 79 percent of men and 86 percent of women respondents said that they had made love for more than fifteen minutes the last time they made love. Twenty percent of men and 15 percent of women said they had made love for more than an *hour* the last time they made love (Michael et al., *Sex in America,* p. 136 table). This does not indicate the actual amount of time they had intercourse, but that figure is no doubt a far cry from Kinsey's dismal findings on the brevity of American lovemaking fifty years ago.

3. The study was based on information gathered from 805 professional nurses, of whom 42.7 percent were multi-orgasmic. The research was reported in *Psychology Today* (vol. 25, no. 4 [July-August, 1992]: 14).

4. A medical-supply company has now developed a biofeedback computer that uses a tampon-shaped probe that can be inserted into the vagina to tell women the strength of their contractions. This small computer costs over one thousand dollars, but all you really need is an inexpensive stone egg, such as Taoist women have used for millennia, to strengthen your entire vagina.

5. The Eastern sexual traditions have long recognized that women can ejaculate. Over the last twenty years, female ejaculation has been confirmed in the laboratory (see Ladas et al., *The G-Spot*), videotaped, bottled, and tested. Although its exact origin and function are unclear, chemical analysis of female ejaculatory fluid suggests that it is similar to male ejaculatory fluid (see chapter 4).

6. Mead concluded that without the cultural expectation of orgasm, the Arapash women were actually not experiencing orgasm. There is another explanation: Arapash women may also have been experiencing what we in the West in our laboratories would call orgasm, without calling it orgasm. This may also be the case with many Western women, as Lonnie Barbach has pointed out.

7. Barbach, *For Each Other*, p. 71.

CHAPTER SEVEN: YANG AND YANG

1. Tannahill, *Sex in History*, p. 179.
2. Stephen T. Chang, *The Tao of Sexology,* p. 62.

CHAPTER EIGHT: BEFORE YOU CALL THE PLUMBER

1. *The Secrets of the Jade Chamber,* quoted in Jolan Chang, *The Tao of Love and Sex,* p. 79.
2. Tanagho and McAninch, *Smith's General Urology* (Collins et al., 1983; Legros, Mormont, and Servais, 1978; Montague et al., 1979; Spark, White, and Connolly, 1980), p. 700.

3. There are treatments such as vacuum constriction devices, intracavernous injection of vasodilators, and penile prostheses that will allow many men with organic sexual problems to still have erections.

4. Accounts of penis enlargement are anything but new. In his classic seventeenth-century Chinese novel, *The Carnal Prayer Mat,* Li Yu describes the protagonist's surgical implantation of a dog's penis to add to his natural endowment. Whether this is a factual story or the author's fancy, it is quite possible that there were Chinese physicians who, not unlike some of today's plastic surgeons, were motivated more by money than by medicine. There were also no doubt men, then as now, who were willing to go under the knife in the hope that they could increase their "manhood."

5. The Brauers also cite one controlled study in England in 1975 that reported apparent permanent increases in penile length and width after men did specific exercises.

6. Niels Skakkebaek's research and Louis Guilette's congressional "testimony" were reported in a *Newsweek* article titled "The Estrogen Complex" (March 21, 1994, p. 76).

7. Tanagho and McAninch, *Smith's General Urology,* p. 677.

CHAPTER NINE: MAKING LOVE FOR A LIFETIME

1. Kinsey et al., *Sexual Behavior in the Human Male,* p. 226.

2. Winn and Newton, 1982. Quoted in Katchadourian, *Fundamentals of Human Sexuality,* p. 385.

3. More than 75 percent of the men aged sixty-one to seventy-one were engaging in coitus at least once a month; also, 37 percent of those aged sixty-one to sixty-five and 28 percent of those aged sixty-six to seventy-one had coitus at least once a week. Among those aged sixty-six to seventy-one, only 10 percent of the men (and 5 percent of the women) claimed to have *no* sexual desire. *Consumer Reports* survey of 4,246 men and women. Reported in Katchadourian, *Fundamentals of Human Sexuality,* p. 385.

4. Dunn and Trost, "Male Multiple Orgasms," p. 385.

5. Masters and Johnson, *Human Sexual Inadequacy.* Boston: Little, Brown, 1970.

6. Ann Landers conducted a survey of 141,000 men and women between the ages of seventeen and ninety-three. She found that 82 percent of the people surveyed felt that sex after marriage was much less pleasurable. Quoted in Brauer and Brauer, *The ESO Ecstasy Program,* p. 4.

7. Zilbergeld, *The New Male Sexuality,* p. 375.

8. Kinsey et al., *Sexual Behavior in the Human Male,* p. 579.

9. *Time,* February 15, 1993, p. 39. Helen Fisher, the author of *Anatomy of Love,* states with regard to endorphins, "That is one reason why it feels so horrible when we're abandoned or a lover dies. We don't have our daily hit of narcotics."

10. Chuck Norris, *The Secret of Inner Strength* (Charter, 1989), pp. 163–64, quoted in Zilbergeld, *The New Male Sexuality,* p. 573. Bernie Zilbergeld's book has a superb discussion of what men can do for their sons. He discusses

the issue at much greater length than we can here and makes especially help-ful suggestions for fathers who are trying to overcome years of estrangement and absence, and for divorced fathers.

11. According to the Tao, contraction and expansion, the pulsation that we call orgasm, is happening in the universe all the time. This is why orgasm is often felt as an "oceanic" experience that makes us feel like we are at one with the universe. The reason we feel "at one" is that we are.

PARTNER EXERCISES

HEALING TAO BOOKS AND INSTRUCTORS

The sexual practices described in this book are part of a complete system of physical, emotional, and spiritual development called the Healing Tao, which is based on the practical teachings of the Taoist tradition. Following is a list of other Healing Tao books written by Mantak Chia.

HEALING TAO BOOKS

Awaken Healing Energy Through the Tao

Awaken Healing Light of the Tao (with Maneewan Chia)

Bone Marrow Nei Kung: Iron Shirt Chi Kung III (with Maneewan Chia)

Chi Nei Tsang: Internal Organ Chi Massage (with Maneewan Chia)

Chi Self-Massage: The Taoist Way of Rejuvenation

Fusion of the Five Elements I (with Maneewan Chia)

Healing Love Through the Tao: Cultivating Female Sexual Energy (with Maneewan Chia)

The Inner Structure of Tai Chi: Tai Chi Kung I (with Juan Li)

Iron Shirt Chi Kung I: Internal Organs Exercise

Taoists Secrets of Love: Cultivating Male Sexual Energy (with Michael Winn)

Taoist Ways to Transform Stress into Vitality

To order Healing Tao books, audiocassettes, or videotapes, write, call, or fax the Healing Tao Center, 1205 O'Neill Highway, Dunmore, PA 18512 (tel. 717-348-4310; fax 717-348-4313).

HEALING TAO INSTRUCTORS

There are over three hundred Healing Tao instructors throughout the world who teach classes and workshops in various practices, from Sexual Kung Fu to Tai-chi and *chi-kung*. For more information about instructors and workshops in your area, contact the Healing Tao Center, 1205 O'Neill Highway, Dunmore, PA 18512 (tel. 717-348-4310; fax 717-348-4313), or the International Healing Tao Center, 274 Moo 7, Laung Nua, Doi Saket, Chiang Mai 50220, Thailand (tel. 66-53-495-596; fax 66-53-495-852).

Anand, Margo. *The Art of Sexual Ecstasy: The Path of Sacred Sexuality for Western Lovers.* Los Angeles: Jeremy P. Tarcher, 1989.

Barbach, Lonnie. *For Each Other: Sharing Sexual Intimacy.* New York: Anchor Books, 1983.

Belzer, E., B. Whipple, and W. Moger. "On Female Ejaculation." *Journal of Sex Research* 20 (1984): 403–406.

Brauer, Alan P., and Donna J. Brauer. *ESO: The New Promise of Pleasure for Couples in Love.* New York: Warner Books, 1983.

———. *The ESO Ecstasy Program.* New York: Warner Books, 1990.

Chang, Jolan. *The Tao of Love and Sex: The Ancient Chinese Way to Ecstasy.* New York: E. P. Dutton, 1977.

———. *The Tao of the Loving Couple: True Liberation Through the Tao.* New York: E. P. Dutton, 1983.

Chang, Stephen T. *The Tao of Sexology: The Book of Infinite Wisdom.* San Francisco: Tao Publishing, 1986.

Chu, Valentin. *The Yin-Yang Butterfly: Ancient Chinese Sexual Secrets for Western Lovers.* Los Angeles: Jeremy P. Tarcher, 1993.

Dunn, M., and J. Trost. "Male Multiple Orgasms: A Descriptive Study." *Archives of Sexual Behavior* 18, no. 5 (1989): 377–87.

Federation of Feminist Women's Health Centers. *A New View of a Woman's Body.* West Hollywood, CA: Feminist Health Press, 1991.

Gray, John. *Mars and Venus in the Bedroom.* New York: HarperCollins Publishers, 1995.

Hartman, William, and Marilyn Fithian. *Any Man Can: The Multiple Orgasmic Technique for Every Loving Man.* New York: St. Martin's Press, 1984.

Hite, Shere. *The Hite Report: A Nationwide Study of Female Sexuality.* New York: Macmillan, 1976.

The Institute for Advanced Study of Human Sexuality. *The Complete Guide to Safer Sex.* Edited by Ted McIlvenna. Fort Lee, NJ: Barricade Books, 1992.

Katchadourian, Herant. *Fundamentals of Human Sexuality.* 4th ed. New York: Holt, Rinehart and Winston, 1985.

Keesling, Barbara. *How to Make Love All Night and Drive a Woman Wild.* New York: HarperCollins Publishers, 1994.

Kinsey, Alfred C., Wardell B. Pomeroy, and Clyde E. Martin. *Sexual Behavior in the Human Male.* Philadelphia: W. B. Saunders, 1948.

Kinsey, Alfred C., Wardell B. Pomeroy, Clyde E. Martin, and Paul H. Gebhard. *Sexual Behavior in the Human Female.* Philadelphia, W. B. Saunders, 1953.

Ladas, Alice Kahn, Beverly Whipple, and John D. Perry. *The G Spot and Other Recent Discoveries About Human Sexuality.* New York: Holt, Rinehart, and Winston, 1982. Dell Paperbacks, 1983.

Masters, William H., Virginia E. Johnson, and Robert C. Kolodny. *Masters and Johnson on Sex and Human Loving.* Boston: Little, Brown and Company, 1986. (Revised edition of *Human Sexuality* [2d ed., 1985].)

Michael, Robert T., John H. Gagnon, Edward O. Laumann, and Gina Kolata. *Sex in America.* Boston: Little, Brown and Company, 1994.

Reich, Wilhelm. *The Function of the Orgasm.* Translated by Vincent R. Carfagno. New York: Farrar, Straus and Giroux, 1973.

Reid, Daniel P. *The Tao of Health, Sex, and Longevity.* New York: Simon & Schuster, 1989.

Robbins, M. B., and G. D. Jensen. "Multiple Orgasms in Males." *Journal of Sex Research* 14 (1978): 21–26.

Schipper, Kristofer. *The Taoist Body.* Berkeley: University of California Press, 1993.

Silverstein, Charles, and Felice Picano. *The New Joy of Gay Sex.* New York: HarperCollins Publishers, 1992.

Stoppard, Miriam. *The Magic of Sex.* New York: Dorling Kindersley, 1991.

Tanagho, Emil A., and Jack W. McAninch, eds. *Smith's General Urology*, 13th ed. Norwalk, CT: Appleton & Lange, 1992.

Tannahill, Reay. *Sex in History.* Rev. ed. London: Cardinal, 1989.

Wile, Douglas. *Art of the Bedchamber: The Chinese Sexual Yoga Classics Including Women's Solo Meditation Texts.* Albany: State University of New York Press, 1992.

Zilbergeld, Bernie. *The New Male Sexuality.* New York: Bantam Books, 1992.